AMBULATORY SURGICAL CENTERS
Development and Management

Thomas R. O'Donovan, Ph.D.

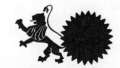

Aspen Systems Corporation
Germantown, Maryland
1976

"This publication is designed to provide accurate and authoritative information in regard to the Subject Matter covered. It is sold with the understanding that the publisher is not engaged in rendering legal, accounting, or other professional service. If legal advice or other expert assistance is required, the services of a competent professional person should be sought."
From a Declaration of Principles jointly adopted by a Committee of the American Bar Association and a Committee of Publishers and Associations.

Library of Congress Catalog Card Number: 76-15767
ISBN:0-912862-21-1

Printed in the United States of America.
1 2 3 4 5

CONTRIBUTORS

Barbara Bregande
President
Innovative Programs, Inc.
20940 N. W. Miami Ct.
Miami, Florida 33169

L. Donald Bridenbaugh, MD
Associate Director
Department of Anesthesiology
Mason Clinic
Virginia Mason Hospital
1118 Ninth Ave.
Seattle, Washington 98101

Magruder C. Donaldson, MD
Bureau of Quality Assurance
Health Services Administration
Department of Health, Education,
    and Welfare
Rockville, Maryland 20852

Marie Erbstoeszer
Health Care Consultant
217 E. Division St.
Mt. Vernon, Washington 98273

Jeffry C. Faine
Administrator
Ambulatory Surgical Facility
4470 Sheridan St.
Hollywood, Florida 33021

Alfred S. Frobese, MD
Director of Surgery
Abington Memorial Hospital
1245 Highland Ave.
Abington, Pennsylvania 19001

Michael J. Goran, MD
Director
Bureau of Quality Assurance
Health Services Administration
Department of Health, Education,
    and Welfare
Rockville, Maryland 20852

Douglas D. Hawthorne
Assistant Administrator
Presbyterian Hospital of Dallas
8200 Walnut Hill Lane
Dallas, Texas 75231

iii

J. Barry Johnson
Administrator
Phoenix Baptist Hospital
6025 N. 20th Ave.
Phoenix, Arizona 85015

M. Robert Knapp, MD
President
Minor Surgery Center® of Wichita
1128 So. Clifton
Wichita, Kansas 67218

Rodney Lamb
Administrator
Santa Barbara Cottage Hospital
Pueblo at Bath St.
Santa Barbara, California 93105

J. D. Manes, MD
Medical Director
Holy Cross Hospital of Calgary
2210 2nd St., S.W.
Calgary, Alberta, Canada T2S 1S6

John C. McCabe
Chief Administrative Officer and
   President
Blue Cross and Blue Shield of
   Michigan
600 Lafayette E.
Detroit, Michigan 48226

Thomas R. O'Donovan, Ph.D
Administrator
Mt. Carmel Mercy Hospital
6071 W. Outer Drive
Detroit, Michigan 48235 `

John D. Porterfield, MD
Director
Joint Commission on Accreditation
   of Hospitals
875 No. Michigan Ave.
Chicago, Illinois 60611

Robert Raatjes
Assistant Administrator for Fiscal
   Affairs
Phoenix Baptist Hospital
6025 N. 20th Ave.
Phoenix, Arizona 85015

Wallace A. Reed, MD
Surgicenter®
1040 E. McDowell Rd.
Phoenix, Arizona 85006

Allen Weltmann
Partner
Coopers & Lybrand
1251 Avenue of the Americas
New York, New York 10020

Bradley W. Yost
Director
Health Care Policy
Blue Cross Association
840 N. Lake Shore Drive
Chicago, Illinois 60611

This book is dedicated to:

My wife, Gayle, and our children Patrick, Lynda, and Julie

and to

The entire Mt. Carmel family.

Author royalties of this book are being donated to the Mt. Carmel Mercy Hospital Guild for their pledge toward our new Pediatric Psychiatry inpatient unit.

Table of Contents

FOREWORD

More than ten years have passed since the concept of ambulatory surgery was reintroduced. It is interesting to note that when the paper by Dr. David Cohen and me was submitted for publication it was, at first, rejected because the idea was considered "contrary to good medical practice."

In many locations, experience over the past ten years of those involved in ambulatory surgery has demonstrated that it is safe, economical, acceptable to patients, saves professional time and releases hospital beds. Yet, 60% of hospitals are unprepared to engage in ambulatory surgery.

Dr. O'Donovan's foresight in organizing and fostering the National Conferences on Ambulatory Surgery has done much to advance good patient care.

This book places the various facets of ambulatory surgery in perspective. To coin a phrase, "it puts it all together." This work deserves careful reading and thoughtful consideration.

It has been an honor and privilege to be associated with the author over the past years in his efforts to improve patient care through the proper application of ambulatory surgery.

John B. Dillon, MD
Professor Emeritus
Department of Anesthesiology
UCLA School of Medicine
Los Angeles, Calif.

Koloa, Kauai
Hawaii

PREFACE

This book discusses the steps that are needed to create or expand a formal program of Ambulatory Surgery in both hospital units and independently operated facilities. The broad issues affecting the quality and performance of ambulatory surgery are also presented.*

The entire gamut of ambulatory surgery is covered in sufficient depth to be a useful handbook to all interested health care professionals. Several case studies are analyzed to show the detailed approaches taken by health care facilities in establishing and maintaining viable programs of ambulatory surgery. Some of the issues discussed are: whether or not additional surgery facilities are needed for the present load, or if hospitals and/or independently operated facilities have to create or expand ambulatory surgical facilities; who should do it, the hospital or the independents; is "peaceful coexistence" possible; the cost implications; how such units can be established—staffing, organization; role of the surgeon versus the role of the anesthesiologist; reimbursement; which surgery is most amenable to ambulatory treatment; should centers be organized on a profit or nonprofit basis; how to obtain a certificate of need; and how should a hospital institute such a program.

Ambulatory surgery will place a great challenge on the traditional hospital system. It has often been said that hospitals charge higher prices than necessary for ambulatory surgery in order to finance the more complicated operative inpatient procedures, such as kidney transplants. If a large number of present inpatients are converted to outpatients, this will increase the average length of stay for such hospitals. If their backlog is high enough, they will continue with a high occupancy but with a greater need for more intensive nursing, which will increase overall personnel costs. Despite these consequences, the result will be

*Most of the chapters have been developed from major papers presented at recent conferences on ambulatory surgery directed by the American Academy of Medical Administrators in the United States.

a greater utilization of hospital resources. If the creation of ambulatory surgery will result in the construction of fewer acute beds, the American health care system will save millions of dollars.

The typical cases for ambulatory surgery are nonemergent, noninfected and elective. Performed under general anesthesia, these procedures take less than an hour and require less than a two-hour stay in the recovery room.

FACT: As of 1976, 60% of our nation's hospitals have no program of ambulatory surgery.

FACT: Ambulatory surgery reduces the average total cost per patient treated in a hospital.

FACT: If hospitals establish a program of ambulatory surgery, and if this removes some of the inpatient stays (without replacing them with new patients), ambulatory surgery *for some hospitals can decrease occupancy* and create an adverse financial impact.

The question arises whether all hospitals should embark upon or enlarge a program of ambulatory surgery. Ambulatory surgery should be tailored to the needs of the community, which are often expressed by the degree of acceptance from patients and physicians. In most hospitals no ambulatory surgery program exists, yet in other hospitals over 20% of all operative procedures are done on an ambulatory basis. Experts have told us that nearly 30% of all surgery performed in the U.S. could be performed on an ambulatory basis. From a fiscal standpoint it is challenging to note that if 30% of the surgery performed in the U.S. could be performed on an ambulatory basis, and if there were no backlog to fill the gap, bed vacancies could result. This could place many fiscal challenges upon hospitals that are considering ambulatory surgery.

Nevertheless, our nation's health care system must seek reasonable ways to contain costs. Reducing inpatient stays is very important *even when low occupancy exists.* Ambulatory surgery should not be reserved only for the hospitals with high occupancy.

There are enormous *long-run* dollar cost savings that can result from ambulatory surgery. Anytime a situation exists when the length of stay of a large number of operative procedures decreases, the opportunity for cost reduction arises and the need to build fewer new beds can occur. As our nation's population expansion continues upward, even though more slowly now, new inpatient beds will be needed in certain areas, although a smaller and smaller number will be needed if more than 20% of all future elective surgery is performed on a "same-day" basis.

Much could be written about the financial importance of reducing a particular patient's hospitalization period for a hernia, for example, from six days to three days. This example could be expanded upon over an enormous range. Professional Standards Review Organizations (PSROs) will have a major impact. But we are talking about reducing many operative procedures to *zero* days. In such instances, special programs need to be established. The fact is that the patient who is discharged the day he arrives requires a wholly different system than the inpatient admission. Systems of patient charges are different, as are space facilities, planning, admitting, pre-op, post-op and discharge. All these areas create fine points of distinction from inpatients simply because the patient arrives the day of surgery instead of one or more days before, and is discharged the same day instead of at a future date.

Ambulatory surgical centers are appropriate for any size hospital. Those hospitals with existing programs which are discussed in this book range in bed-size capacity.

Abington Memorial Hospital 469 beds
Santa Barbara Cottage Hospital 407 beds
Presbyterian Baptist Hospital 170 beds
Holy Cross Hospital 533 beds
Virginia Mason Hospital 287 beds
Mt. Carmel Mercy Hospital 559 beds

Thomas R. O'Donovan
Mt. Carmel Mercy Hospital

August 1976

Acknowledgements

I should like to express deep appreciation to the American Academy of Medical Administrators and to all the faculty members who made such an outstanding contribution to the literature on this key issue in health care delivery.

Words cannot express the gratitude I have to the person that made this book possible, Sister Mary Leila, R.S.M., Executive Director of Mt. Carmel Mercy Hospital and President of the American Academy of Medical Administrators from 1973 to 1976. Day-to-day hospital dynamics generally preclude the time needed to write articles and books, but not so with the leadership and encouragement provided to me by Sister Leila, the best boss in the world.

PART I
MASTER PLAN OF
AMBULATORY SURGERY

The purpose of Part I is to develop a conceptual framework for the concept of ambulatory surgery. The first four chapters are original papers by the author which discuss the definition, historical development, and scope of the subject. The overall model of ambulatory surgery is presented, using three different hospital models and the model of the independently operated surgical facility. Each one is described, with the complete range of the advantages and disadvantages. A special section foiuses on the major conclusions of ambulatory surgery: where we stand today in the U.S. after a full examination of the literature. At this point some key research-oriented hypotheses are presented.

Chapter 4 describes the mechanics of ambulatory surgery; how a facility can establish prices; should a blanket charging mechanism be established; and the implications of using different color-coded charge tickets to distinguish ambulatory surgery from inpatient surgery. Specific steps in setting up a formal program of ambulatory surgery are outlined as well as the problems that must be overcome. The main objective of this chapter is to provide an extensive treatment of the major cost features of ambulatory surgery. One major shortcoming in the existing literature on the subject is the conclusions relating to cost that have no factual documentation.

A complete comparative treatment of the cost issues for hospitals and independent facilities is presented.

The text shows how ambulatory surgery can, under certain circumstances, increase both total costs and unit costs. Describing the impact of ambulatory surgery on short-run and long-run community costs, the chapter explores the following questions: do independently operated surgical facilities reduce the cost of community health care delivery?; and, in a cost-based reimbursement system, do hospitals that establish formal programs of ambulatory surgery reduce community costs more than the independent facilities?

1

In Chapter 5 Barbara J. Bregande, develops some major concepts in the design and organizational flow of ambulatory surgery units, contributing a substantial addition to the literature.

Chapter 1
Major Concepts And Definitions

Thomas R. O'Donovan

This book is devoted to formal, organized programs of elective ambulatory surgery in which patients arrive and are discharged the same day. Such patients are operated on, mostly under general anesthesia, in a hospital, near a hospital, or a hospital satellite, or in a nonhospital, independently operated facility.[1] We are *not* referring to the millions of "same-day" procedures performed in doctors' offices throughout the country. We are not describing surgery that is performed in a hospital's outpatient department by house staff under local anesthesia; nor are we relating to the thousands of operative procedures performed on patients in emergency departments throughout the U.S.

Across the country, major health care changes are taking place to improve the level of patient care, reduce duplication of medical services, and reduce or contain costs of health care delivery. One of the major innovations is ambulatory surgery which is sweeping North America.[2]

According to the American Hospital Association (AHA), "Many types of minor surgery do not require overnight hospitalization. Therefore hospitals must plan and provide outpatient surgical facilities so that, whenever appropriate, surgery can be performed on an outpatient basis, thereby reducing costs to the patient, the hospital, and the community, and assuring optimum use of inpatient beds."[3]

There is no question of the importance of ambulatory surgery in medical care in modern day America. Ambulatory surgery should be integrated within the community-wide plan for health services. Nonduplication of facilities must be documented and a balance should be attained between quality care and cost containment. Ambulatory surgery can provide more hospital beds for seriously ill patients and reduce waiting time for elective surgery. This trend is occurring because of new techniques in anesthesia and in control of bleeding, and other health safeguards, as well as physician and patient acceptance.[4] Some
Some pediatric physicians experienced in ambulatory surgery have pre-

3

dicted that within five years, over half of all pediatric surgery will be done on an ambulatory basis.[5]

Many new diagnostic testing procedures are appearing in the health care delivery field. With the advent of these sophisticated diagnostic testing procedures, many patients who would normally have to be hospitalized for one or several days can now be evaluated as outpatients. In fact, one of the strong arguments in favor of the Computerized Tomography (CT) scanner is its impact on reducing, or even avoiding, hospitalization. According to Eugene E. Duda, M.D., "For patients, this machine offers significant advances in convenience, speed, and comfort. Prior to its installation, our patients were subjected to one or more diagnostic techniques that required hospitalization and involved some degree of discomfort. The three most common tests were pneumoencephalography, injecting air into the spaces in and around the brain; angiography, injecting opaque dye into the blood vessels of the brain; and radioisotope scanning, detecting abnormal accumulations of radioactive tracers in the brain. The first two procedures are more expensive than the CT examination, and require hospitalization."[6]

Ambulatory surgical patients often return to work sooner than if they had been hospitalized for the same procedure. An increasing number of hospital programs in ambulatory surgery are emerging, and the range of procedures is large.[7] Each case depends upon the judgment of the attending physician, as well as on the desires of the patient, the type of insurance coverage, and access to short-stay surgical facilities.

HISTORICAL DEVELOPMENT OF AMBULATORY SURGERY[8]

Although a great deal of attention is currently focused on ambulatory surgery, it really is not a new idea. Published reports describing ambulatory surgery go back as far as the beginning of the century. One of the earliest reports was that of J.H. Nichol, M.D., of Glasgow.[9] At a meeting of the British Medical Association in 1909, he reported on 7,320 operations which he had performed on ambulatory patients at the Royal Glasgow Hospital for Children. The ambulatory surgery results were reportedly as successful as those for children who were treated as inpatients. Another major report was made by Gertrude Herzfeld of Edinburgh in 1938.[10] When a series of over 1,000 hernia repairs was performed on children, with many of the operations done on an outpatient basis, using a general anesthetic, good results were reported.

In spite of these early successes, ambulatory surgery did not receive much attention in the field of medicine for a number of years. The lack of published reports should not, however, be interpreted to mean that ambulatory surgery was not practiced. Many physicians, oral surgeons, and podiatrists apparently have performed a variety of surgical procedures in this way throughout the years. With the increasing specialization of medicine there may however, have been an inclination to bring surgery to the hospitals where the surgical specialsts were practicing. Thus, there may have been an ebb and flow in the reported utilization of the practice of ambulatory surgery.

In the early 1960s a number of factors caused an increased interest in ambulatory surgery. A major factor was the development of new anesthetics and anesthetic techniques which made ambulatory surgery safer and more acceptable to physicians. ("Improved anesthetics are a major factor in the spread of same-day surgery units, doctors say. Today's fast acting anesthetics, explains Dr. Penta, 'wear off faster and leave fewer after-effects.' ") Furthermore, as the practice of surgery evolved, surgeons wanted many of their patients to move around sooner. Since many hospitals were then experiencing a high demand for inpatient beds, ambulatory surgery was welcomed as a mechanism for freeing up these badly needed beds for patients who were seriously ill. Ambulatory surgery was also viewed as providing potential conveniences for both physicians and patients, and thus the concept gained further acceptance. Finally, the potential for cost savings or containment, since patients were not hospitalized for two or three days, also caused increased interest in ambulatory surgery.

This interest in ambulatory surgery has spread rapidly. John Dillon, M.D., and David Cohen, M.D., at the University of California in Los Angeles (UCLA) established a hospital-based program. The program at UCLA has been very successful and has provided excellent guidelines for subsequent programs.[12] Another early program in the United States was the come-and-go surgery unit at George Washington University, which opened in March, 1966.[13]

More recently, freestanding facilities for ambulatory surgery have developed. Probably the earliest recognized freestanding surgical center was the Dudley Street Ambulatory Surgical Center in Providence, Rhode Island, which opened in December, 1968.[14] It was founded by Charles Hill, M.D., and four associates. In 1970, Wallace Reed, M.D., and John Ford, M.D., of Phoenix, Arizona established the Surgicenter®, a non-hospital-based ambulatory surgical facility.[15] The Surgicenter® has gained broad acceptance and has become well known as a model for other developing freestanding facilities.

Federal initiative has also been instrumental in generating interest in ambulatory surgery. Public Law 92-603 provides for the establishment of Professional Standards Review Organizations (PSROs).

When the PSROs are functional, they will be required to certify that Medicare and Medicaid patients are being cared for in the least complex and least costly manner appropriate to the medical problem. The likelihood of a National Health Insurance Program has also drawn attention to ambulatory surgery. It is anticipated that such an insurance program may increase the demand for all health services. If so, ambulatory surgery is viewed as helping to reduce the demand for hospital beds.

The International Perspective

As noted above, the extensive use of ambulatory surgery was first reported by physicians in the United Kingdom. At present this concept is widely received and practiced under the British National Health System. Numerous recent reports cite the value of ambulatory surgery to both physicians and patients.[16] The demand for hospital beds is very high in Britain, where nonemergent surgical cases reportedly must wait for an extensive period prior to getting scheduled for admission. Thus, the provision of ambulatory services is viewed as saving both time and money, while still providing high quality medical care.

While a complete review of the international literature has not been pursued, a few additional examples will illustrate that interest in ambulatory surgery is widespread. Canadian publications have cited their views of the advantages of providing ambulatory surgery services.[17] Potential cost savings and convenience to patients, especially children, were key positive points. Gien, a South African physician, has reported on 5,321 ambulatory surgery cases performed between 1965-1971. The author cites the savings of dollars to the patient, the increased productivity of nursing staff and better utilization of the limited number of hospital beds as prime factors supporting the provision of ambulatory surgery.[18]

Early Ambulation

Paul T. Lahti, M.D., has performed some valuable work that relates to the general concept and theory of ambulatory surgery. His work relates to early ambulation of patients, which has an obvious application to ambulatory surgery.[19] Dr. Lahti has published documented evidence based on over 1,000 consecutive cases of patients relating to early ambulation after postoperative discharge. He has updated the original study reported in 1970, which now includes data on over 2,000 patients. He points out that in the past 30 years the period of hospitalization necessary after surgery has decreased steadily.

Some of Dr. Lahti's observations and conclusions are: (1) If without surgery a healthy person were put to bed for a week and given narcotics at various intervals, it would take several weeks for recovery from this experience; (2) It is now possible and desirable to discharge the majority of surgical patients on the first or second postoperative day; (3) The usual patient entering the hospital for major surgery is frightened of the unknown, and when he awakens from the anesthetic, his fears are brought to the surface so that any minor discomfort is magnified into real pain; and (4) Narcotics only prolong the recovery, whereas the patient who knows that he will be up and about the afternoon of surgery and home the day after surgery is relaxed, not fearful, and requires much less postoperative medication. Infants and young children have not been conditioned to being ill following surgery, and as a result, they usually are not.

Some of the examples of surgery noted in the report by Dr. Lahti include unilateral and bilaterial inguinal hernia, appendectomy, ligation and stripping of saphenous veins, hemorrhoidectomy, excision of pilonidal cyst, excision of breast tumor, simple and radical mastectomy, thyroidectomy, and cholecystectomy. For an adult usually one or two doses of 50 mg of Demerol is sufficient. If a patient is reluctant to go home, it is helpful to explain that as soon as the need for hospitalization ceases he is much better off at home. It is important, however, that he knows of the small but very real incidence of postoperative complications caused by being inactive and in a hospital. The patient is advised to bathe daily and to wash over the sutures with soap and water. Patients are advised that they may be up and about as much as they desire, and resume normal activities, including driving. Many patients return to work before the sutures are removed.

At a time of rapidly rising costs, early postoperative discharge of patients offers a method of decreasing hospital costs by 30%. Certain studies show that American's average length of stay is approximately 7 to 8 days. In the data reported by Dr. Lahti all patients were discharged by the seventh postoperative day; 75 of the first 1,114 patients were discharged by the second day. In the updated study based on 2,000 patients these figures tended to remain about the same. According to Dr. Lahti, there are no valid reasons for keeping patients in the hospital any longer than necessary to recover from the anesthetic in the usual case. The patient's fear that something might go wrong if he goes home can now be changed to *something might go wrong* if he stays in the *hospital.* His conclusion is that although it is difficult to overcome the traditions and habits of the past, the results are certainly worth the effort.

The lessons are therefore clear: if patients spend a shorter length of stay in the hospital, the result is more effective utilization of health care delivery resources. This, in turn, can help stem the tide of escalating hospital costs.

Notes

1. In 1961, Butterworth Hospital in Grand Rapids, Michigan, was a major pioneer in the hospital approach to a formal program of ambulatory surgery.

2. Thomas R. O'Donovan, "The Dynamics of Ambulatory Surgery," *Hospital Administration*, Winter 1975, p. 27-29.

3. *Hospitals, JAHA,* August 1, 1973, p. 132.

4. D. D. Cohen and J. B. Dillon, "Anesthesia for Outpatient Surgery," *Journal of the American Medical Association,* Vol. 196, January 27, 1966, pp. 11-14; A Doenicke, J. Kugler, and M. Laub, "Evaluation of Recovery and 'Streetfitness' by EEG and Psychodiagnostic Tests After Anesthesia," *Canadian Anesthetists's Society Journal,* Vol. 14, 1967, p. 567; A. Fahy and M. Marshall, "Postanesthetic Morbidity in Outpatients," *British Journal of Anaesthesiology,* Vol. 41, 1969, p. 433; and K. M. Janis, "Hospital-Based Outpatient Anesthesia Service: Organization and Management," *The Hospital Medical Staff,* February 1973, pp. 12-16.

5. D. T. Cloud, et. al., "The Surgicenter: A Fresh Concept in Outpatient Pediatric Surgery," *Journal of Pediatric Surgery,* Vol. 7, April 1972, pp. 206-212; H. T. Davenport et al., "Day Surgery for Children," *Canadian Medical Association Journal,* Vol. 105, 1971, p. 498; " 'One-Day-Stay' Plan for Pediatric Patients: Hospital of the Albert Einstein College of Medicine," *Medical World News,* Vol. 12, 1971, p. 48B; C. L. Rosenberg, "Short-Stay Surgical Center for Your Patients" (Surgicenter,® Phoenix, Arizona), *Medical Economics,* Vol. 48, 1971, p. 114; and B. Tisdale, "Not for Admission—Day Care Surgery for Children," *Canadian Nurse,* Vol. 68, December 1972, pp. 35-39.

6. Gregg W. Downey, "A Scanner for Every Hospital?" *Modern Healthcare,* February 1976, pp. 16s-16w.

7. *Wall Street Journal,* Vol. 54, No. 1, January 4, 1974, p. 15.

8. The following extract is from Marie Erbstoeszer, "Ambulatory Surgery Criteria and Standards Monograph," University of Washington for the Health Resources Administration, Department of Health, Education, and Welfare. Contract No.: HRA 106-74-56, 1975.

9. J. H. Nichol, "Paper presented at the British Medical Association Meeting," *British Medical Journal,* Vol. 2, 1909, p. 753.

10. G. Herzfeld, "Hernia in Infancy," *American Journal of Surgery,* Vol. 39, 1938, pp. 422-429.

11. *Wall Street Journal,* p. 15.

12. Cohen and Dillon, pp. 98-100.

13. M. L. Levy and C. S. Coakley, "Survey of In and Out Surgery—The First Year," *Southern Medical Journal,* Vol. 61, September 1968, pp. 995-998.

14. "Outpatient Surgery," *Hospital Administration Currents,* Vol. 16, April 1972, pp. 1-4.

15. J. Ford and W. Reed, "The Surgicenter®—An Innovation in the Delivery and Cost of Medical Care," *Arizona Medicine,* Vol. 26, October 1969, pp. 801-804.

16. G. Craig, "Use of Day Beds in Gynaecology," *British Medical Journal,* Vol. 2, June 27, 1970, pp. 786-787; Calnan and P. Martin, "Development and Practice of an Autonomous Minor Surgery Unit in a General Hospital," *British Medical Journal,* Vol. 4, October 9, 1971, pp. 92-96; S. G. Clayton et al., "Shortstay Gynaecology Ward," *The Lancet,* November 27, 1971, pp. 1197-1198; T. H. Berrill, "A Year in the Life of a Surgical Day Unit," *British Medical Association Journal,* Vol. 4, November 11, 1972, pp. 348-349.

17. "Curbing the Costs," editorial, *Canadian Medical Association Journal,* Vol. 107, July 22, 1972, pp. 103-104; B. Tisdale, "Not for Admission," *The Canadian Nurse,* December 1972, pp. 35-39; J. E. Treloar, "An Outpatient Anesthetic Service: Standards and Organization," *Canadian Anaesthetist's Society Journal,* Vol. 14, November 1967, pp. 596-604.

18. I. Gien, "Outpatient Surgery in Day Clinics," *South African Medical Journal,* Vol. 45, December 1971, pp. 1,395-1,397.

19. Paul T. Lahti, "Early Post-Operative Discharge of Patients," *Michigan Medicine,* Vol. 69, No. 17, September 1970, pp. 755-760; also "Early Post-Operative Discharge of Patients from the Hospital," *Surgery,* Vol. 63, March 1968, pp. 410-415.

Chapter 2

The Pros and Cons of Ambulatory Surgery

Thomas R. O'Donovan

We have now provided the conceptual framework for our indepth examination of the process of ambulatory surgery. Our next step is to evaluate the usefulness of such surgery within the U.S. system of health care delivery. Since so much additional surgery could be performed on an "in-and-out basis," it would be helpful to investigate the roadblocks. (An extensive listing of surgical procedures eligible to be performed on an ambulatory basis is found in Appendix C.)

In the past few years the American experience with ambulatory surgery has increased dramatically. Much information can be drawn from this experience, but before definitive conclusions are reached, we recommend that more research be conducted in order to properly document the major advantages and disadvantages.

For example, one of the major advantages often mentioned in the literature is the importance of cost reduction that can occur from having sound ambulatory surgery programs in our nation's hospitals. As Chapter 4 illustrates, cost reduction depends upon the system of reimbursement of hospital costs. If hospital costs are reimbursed on the basis of charges made, rather than costs incurred, entirely different answers can be formulated by tracing the impact of an increase in ambulatory surgery. We also have to look at the importance of community costs, as well as an individual hospital's costs, both in the short-run and in the long-run. This chapter will explore these advantages and many others.

Research is needed on the problems in ambulatory surgery also because proper documentation must be established before sound conclusions in this regard can be ascertained.

At the present time, for example, we have very little data on the degree of patient acceptance of ambulatory surgery, whether or not patients fear it. We have heard patients say that "minor surgery is any surgery performed on the other person; major surgery is all surgery performed on me." Even if data

11

were gathered on the degree of patient acceptance, the conclusions might reflect the nature of the institution and the manner of practice of the physician. Many variables would remain.

For many years, the reimbursement policies of insurance companies placed many roadblocks to the performance of ambulatory surgery in hospitals and in independently operated facilities. For example, there were many instances where outpatient surgery was not reimbursed, forcing the patient to be hospitalized in order to receive coverage. This encouraged patients to request hospitalization rather than pay for their care as outpatients.

Ambulatory surgery can take place in various settings. The most common setting is the hospital, but there are at least three different kinds of hospital-controlled ambulatory surgical centers. One very common type is the program in which the hospital creates a formal ambulatory surgical program by superimposing it upon its existing inpatient care system. In this way, additional operating rooms are not constructed, and the ambulatory patients use the same preop and postop areas, as well as the same admitting areas as inpatients. Another hospital type model is a specially created facility tailormade for ambulatory surgery on the grounds of the hospital. A third hospital model is the satellite, which is the creation of a separate ambulatory surgical facility located some distance from the hospital. The fourth model described in this chapter is the independently operated freestanding ambulatory surgery center. The various advantages and disadvantages of each kind of center is detailed in this chapter.

With the decline in the nation's birthrate in recent years, a rather large number of obstetrical departments have closed; some hospitals have utilized a former obstetrical unit for ambulatory surgery. In Bethesda, Maryland, Suburban Hospital recently closed its obstetrical department and converted the space into a very excellent ambulatory surgical center. According to its administrator, Robin H. Hagaman, the hospital has developed a very active ambulatory surgical service in recent years and, with the consolidation of this activity into the new ambulatory surgical wing, they expect continued growth.

Sometimes ambulatory surgery is performed in emergency departments of hospitals. According to Phalen,

> When outpatient surgical services are provided within the emergency room, the same operating room that is used for minor emergency procedures also is used for minor elective procedures. Constant staffing coverage and nonduplication of facilities are the primary advantages of this arrangement, which has often been used in Canada. On the other hand, the primary disadvantage of providing outpatient surgery in the emergency room is that the patient may not receive the individualized attention that he might otherwise expect. The tense emergency room environment, together with the unpredictable levels

of activity and concomitant allocation of personnel resources, usually results in a poorly functioning outpatient surgery facility.[1]

THE PROS AND CONS OF AMBULATORY SURGERY

Advantages

1. Reduced cost; (at least $100 per procedure); less patient work-up is needed. There are more lab tests given and pharmacy items prescribed for inpatients than for ambulatory surgical patients for the same procedure. There is a definite difference in the scope of medical management of inpatients and ambulatory surgical patients by physicians.
2. More effective use of physicians' time. This tends to be a greater advantage in the independently operated facilities than in hospitals.
3. Reduced bed congestion in busy hospitals.
   a) May make more room for seriously ill patients.
   b) May reduce the need to construct new beds, or at least delay or reduce number of new beds needed in a given community.
4. Patient may return to work a day or two earlier.
5. Less psychological stress of hospitalization. (This is especially true in children.) Easier and more agreeable recovery in the home.
6. Tailormade patient care to meet the needs of the "non-sick." Putting such patients in the hospital for 1-3 days forces them into the hospital's typical inpatient treatment pattern which, by necessity, requires some degree of aloneness, and susceptibility to hospital-acquired infections.
7. Ambulatory surgical patients tend to receive less medication pre-and postoperatively than inpatients because they are under medical supervision a shorter period of time. Research is needed to evaluate this phenomenon.
8. When the hospital is able to attract "new business" by creating or expanding its ambulatory surgery program (from doctors' offices, from new doctors, etc.), it can spread its fixed overall costs, to some extent, over a wider range of services. Many advantages often occur when there is greater use made of anesthesia and OR services, e.g., good anesthesiologists are attracted or remain.

Some Alleged Problems in Ambulatory Surgery

Some of the problems that have come up in discussions of ambulatory surgery include the following:

1. Patient resistance
   a) "My friends always were hospitalized for a D&C, why shoultn't I be?"
   b) "My hospitalization insurance policy pays for inpatient care, and I want all that is coming to me."
   c) "It must be safer to be hospitalized because my doctor never uses the ambulatory surgery program of the hospital.'
2. Physician resistance:
   a) Force of habit; lack of general community acceptance; and lack of immediate availability of care in case sudden complications occur.
   b) Possible increased malpractice danger—depends on area practice because court cases lean heavily on what is "considered common usage." In a community with little ambulatory surgery, a physicain may tend to take a conservative view of "experimentation."
   c) Reduced physician income in inpatient follow-up care.
      1) Not a strong "con" but some critics may make more of this issue than they should.
3. Potentially reduced hospital income. (This point is covered in Chapter 4.)

The Four Basic Models of Ambulatory Surgery Centers

I. HOSPITAL CONTROLLED: USING EXISTING INPATIENT ORS, ADMITTING, PRE- AND POSTOP AREAS. (There are also subvariations, e.g., a hospital could use existing ORs but create separate new admitting section, etc. This increases both efficiency *and* cost. See Appendix H).

Advantages

a) Enables the hospital to establish a capability for ambulatory surgery, with limited capital investment. It is often possible to create this capability without adding admitting clerks or nurses, although in some cases a small amount of additional personnel may be needed, depending on how busy the unit is. Greater "economies of scale" are provided because the new subunit will be part of the overall system.

b) The capability can be established quicker because the basic inpatient facilities already exist, eliminating construction time.

c) Flexibility: If the medical staff, for whatever reason, does not utilize the ambulatory surgery program, no expensive dollar costs have been wasted. (If a complete new unit were constructed and it was not used sufficiently, serious financial problems would result.)

d) This model allows the surgeon to perform more complex surgical procedures which can result in greater utilization of the ambulatory surgical program. For example, if the pathology report on a breast biopsy shows cancer, more definitive surgery can be performed at that time *rather than* waiting until the patient is transferred to the hospital's inpatient area.

Disadvantages

a) Basically, the hospital is organized and established for inpatient care, and when ambulatory surgery, as well as certain other ambulatory programs,[2] are superimposed upon the existing inpatient system, many problem areas can result. Hospital personnel often regard ambulatory surgery patients as second-class citizens. This can lessen the dignity with which patients are treated. When these problems are not solved, utilization of the unit may not reach its full potential.

b) Longer waits for admission for ambulatory surgery because the inpatient admitting people may be busy with work procedures for their inpatients.

c) Some hospitals treat the ambulatory surgery patients who do not have Blue Cross or Medicare insurance differently than inpatients. For example, they may require full cash outlay in advance to pay for outpatient surgery if the patient has a commercial insurance policy, whereas that same patient might have had credit extended as an inpatient for his stay.

d) Higher charges than necessary for ambulatory surgery arising from pricing structures modeled after the inpatient pricing system.

e) Outpatients scheduled for surgery may be bumped by emergency cases taken care of in the operating room. In addition, inpatient surgery generally is awarded priority over ambulatory surgery.

f) Since the preop holding areas and recovery rooms are designed for inpatient surgery, ambulatory surgery patients must be merged in the same areas as sometimes critical inpatients. This can result in unnecessary psychological stress.

g) Often proper waiting room areas for ambulatory surgery patients do not exist. When families of inpatients and outpatients are merged, a negative psychological impact on the families of ambulatory surgery patients can result.

h) Since ambulatory surgery patients *awaken earlier* than inpatients, it often occurs that operating room personnel may not be familiar with the special needs of such ambulatory patients.

i) Possibly a greater incidence of nosocomial infections, especially compared to the freestanding centers.

j) An excessively detailed medical record because of the comprehensive nature of inpatient care.

II. HOSPITAL CONTROLLED: LOCATED ON HOSPITAL GROUNDS IN A SPECIALLY CREATED, NEWLY CONSTRUCTED, OR REMODELED AREA, TAILORMADE FOR AMBULATORY SURGERY. (Similar to the approach taken at Santa Barbara Cottage Hospital, in Santa Barbara, California; see Chapter 7.)

Advantages

a) The biggest advantage is the tendency to relieve the disadvantages enumerated in Model I above. (Although good management could relieve many of the disadvantages of Model I.)

b) Tailormade area for ambulatory surgery to maximize patient care from a physical facilities standpoint more than when area is merged with existing systems). If the area is going to be remodeled rather than newly constructed, care should be taken that a suitable area is selected. For example, if a small area of space is chosen, it may be *insufficient* for a sound ambulatory surgery program.

c) Greater satisfaction on the part of personnel, patients, and physicians, because everything is "tailormade."

d) This type of community service may attract a large share of the market because it may appeal to physicians who are not currently members of the hospital's medical staff.[3]

Disadvantages

a) It can cost too much. A degree of flexibility is lost in this approach because if the unit is not successful, it is not likely that

the space can be utilized for other hospital services without additional capital investment.
   b) Items "c" and "d" under Model I can be disadvantages in Model II as well.
III. HOSPITAL CONTROLLED: THE SATELLITE. Some hospitals háve considered opening a satellite health care facility with ambulatory care as the central thrust, with or without ambulatory surgery. Ambulatory surgery, however, could be the main thrust of such a satellite system. Basically, a satellite ambulatory surgery facility is a freestanding facility in which the unit is located some distance from the hospital. It is created specifically for these purposes and is totally controlled by the hospital. Such satellites can be developed by joint hospital efforts as a "shared service."

Advantages

The same as those in Model II; but, in addition, the medical needs of a specific geographic area can be met on a tailormade basis.

Disadvantages

The same as those outlined in "a" in Model II, plus "a" and "b" described in Model IV.

IV. NONHOSPITAL CONTROLLED: THE INDEPENDENTLY OPERATED FREESTANDING SURGERY CENTER (such as the Phoenix Surgicenter® and the Minor Surgery Center® of Wichita).

Advantages

   a) If a particular community has an absence of ambulatory surgery facilities, or if existing ambulatory surgery facilities are inadequate, for whatever reason, the freestanding units fill a void by providing ambulatory surgery capability to the community.
   b) Lower charges in the freestanding independent units when compared to the hospital charge system.
   c) Tendency for increased patient and physician satisfaction. There appears to be an excessive amount of bureaucratic red tape when patients have ambulatory surgery within the hospital setting. The freestanding units have capitalized on this and many perform admirably in terms of patient care and comfort.

Disadvantages

a) Possible increase in net community cost, under certain circumstances. This is an important issue and research is needed in this area. (See Chapter 4.)

b) Reduced adjacency to hospital emergency back-up facilities. The independents feel that such back-up is not needed for patient safety; therefore, research in this area would be necessary.

c) A noted in the *Business Week* article in Appendix G, Dr. Herbert Notkin is quoted as saying: "Skimming off low-risk, no overhead surgery from hospitals will simply increase the cost of those operations that must be performed in hospitals." The lead-in to the article states that one-day surgery could improve—or maybe wreck—the health care system. Therefore, independently operated ambulatory surgical facilities can present a challenge to hospital delivery of such care. Such a challenge would exist even if hospitals, alone, dramatically embarked on programs of a high incidence of ambulatory surgery.

Notes

[1]James F. Phalen, "Planning a Hospital-Based Outpatient Surgery Program," *Hospital Progress,* Vol. 57, No. 6, June 1976, p. 65.

[2]"In too many hospitals, non-emergency patients who enter the Emergency Department must wait and wait and then wait some more. The lack of privacy and the inadequate separation of waiting and treatment areas offend patient sensibilities, are detrimental to therapy, and detract from the provision of care in a professional manner. The result is unhappy patients and deteriorating community relations." (From: James M. Kiser and Randall L. Kiser, "Gearing Up for the Ambulatory Care Crunch," *Trustee,* December, 1975, p. 19.) Also, see Robin E. MacStravic, "Hospital-Based Ambulatory Care—The Wave of the Future," *Hospital and Health Services Administration,* Winter 1976, p. 60. "Primarily, hospitals have served as a source of inpatient care . . . from the patients' point of view, the hospital has not been the most attractive alternative for ambulatory care."

[3]Phalen, op. cit., p. 65.

Chapter 3
Major Conclusions in Ambulatory Surgery

Thomas R. O'Donovan

The purpose of this chapter is to list major conclusions based on research and study, and to recommend research-oriented hypotheses within the framework of ambulatory surgery.

Throughout the U.S. many patients who undergo surgery and are hospitalized from one to four days could be cared for on a "same day" basis. This concept of ambulatory surgery needs to be recommended by physicians to selected patients who are to undergo certain surgical procedures. From 20% to 40% of all surgery can now be performed without requiring an overnight stay in a hospital.

Acceptance of the concept by physicians is increasing slowly but steadily in spite of the many pressures on them to avoid come-and-go surgery. Some of the factors that deter acceptance include: conservatism, fear of malpractice suits, and a general lack of facilities that help to create the appeal for short-stay surgery. A patient who develops bleeding may be less likely to sue if it happens during hospitalization rather than at home. We would be shocked at the dollar cost of defensive medicine practiced by physicians as a result of the many court judgments in favor of the patient.

As hospitals enlarge or start a coordinated program of ambulatory surgery, they may experience reduced occupancy for the general acute hospital beds unless their surgical and medical patient waiting list is sufficient to cover the reduction. The net effect throughout the country will be a long-run reduction in overall costs of health care delivery. Many hospitals should unquestionably institute or expand such programs, based on need, existence of community facilities, and their own individual capacities. It is interesting to note that if a hospital embarks successfully on a program of ambulatory surgery and has a high backlog, the internal medicine department may want an increased quota of beds, while surgery may want all the "bed savings" for themselves.

The federal government, through Professional Standards Review Organizations (PSROs) will require an increase in ambulatory surgery within our nation's hospitals, although many hospitals are not sufficiently organized or philosophically prepared at the present time.

Independently operated, private, come-and-go surgical facilities increasingly will be competing with hospitals for patients. The new facilities often perform the services in a highly competent and well-organized manner that provides a great deal of satisfaction to the patient. The net effect of such a trend in the large urban centers where hospitals may have excess facilities could be to increase the cost of such delivery of health care to the community because of the present system of cost reimbursement that is so prevalent within the hospital industry.

There is no valid reason why a hospital should necessarily charge more for a surgical procedure on a come-and-go basis than an independently operated freestanding facility. Actually, the hospital should be at an advantage, since the operating suites are already there, the lifesaving support equipment is available, and the element of profit and property taxes necessary in an independent facility can be eliminated.

Unfortunately, the hospital can be placed at a disadvantage by the very agencies (government and Blue Cross) that should be most interested in allowing the existing facilities to be competitive and in eliminating unnecessary duplication of facilities, since such duplication can result only in increasing the total community cost of health care. This disadvantage results from the cost reimbursement mandated by some of the third-party payers, requiring allocation of many items of overhead on a pro-rata basis. The allocation of costs for medical records, housekeeping, maintenance, depreciation, and so forth, may be totally disproportionate to the realities of the added costs incurred, but the *system* often requires this allocation. The net result is that these so-called "costs" force hospitals to charge more for procedures than freestanding facilities. The other side of the coin, and one that is never mentioned, is that by forcing hospitals to over-allocate costs to the ambulatory surgery program, the end result is really a reduction of allocated costs to other departments in the hospital. Hence, the long-run effect well may be to reduce costs in roentgenography, the clinical laboratory, and other areas. This savings gets lost in the immense paperwork jungle of Blue Cross and Medicare, and the focus continues to be on why the hospitals cannot compete with freestanding facilities.

A policy statement adopted by the Board of Trustees of the American Hospital Association (AHA) on May 9, 1973, cautioned that, "The overall impact of providing these services in a communitywide system of health care must be considered, rather than the unit cost per service in the individual facilities." If this factor could be truly and accurately measured, there is no way that any freestanding facility could compete with virtually any existing hospital. The necessary capital expenditures and operating costs at a freestanding facility almost by definition must exceed the *added* costs of a short-stay program in an existing hospital. (See Chapter 4.) The real problem is the inequitable distribution of overhead that appears to put the hospital at a cost disadvantage. (Such overhead is not fully required to establish a hospital ambulatory surgical program.) Blue Cross and Medicare should be told that the reason they are charged $300 by the hospital for a service that the patient can obtain elsewhere for $200, is that *they* (Blue Cross in some states, and Medicare) require hospitals to follow certain cost accounting procedures. It should also be noted that the present Medicare law of the federal government tends to discourage ambulatory surgery in two ways: (1) the existence of a deductible for outpatient surgery of Medicare patients, which may result in many patients pressuring for the surgery to be done as an inpatient; (2) very few independently operated facilities are currently reimbursed under the Medicare program, though this may soon change.

As we approach the 1980's, over one-half of our nation's hospitals have no program of ambulatory surgery. If hospitals open or enlarge ambulatory surgery facilities, they can reduce their present number of inpatient admissions and reduce their percentage of occupancy. But if other strategies are developed, such as new programs, physician recruitment activities, outreach programs, or development of satellites there will be an increase in inpatient stays. We should keep in mind that reducing inpatient stays is an important way of containing costs, even when low occupancy exists.

Quality care is vital. In short-stay surgery you are dealing with *elective* procedures on patients who aren't sick. If death or any serious consequence occurs there is some doubt that the ambulatory surgery unit has a right to exist. The job must be done properly, day-in and day-out.

Hospitals can do the job if such a priority objective is established. They have the facilities and personnel. All it takes is managerial expertise—something that the Phoenix Surgicenter® has had since its inception. In fact, the contribution of Drs. Reed and Ford may be considered one of the great medical landmarks in health care delivery. There is no doubt that the Phoenix Surgicenter® is a sterling example of independently operated freestanding come-and-go surgical facilities. Only time will tell how many other independently operated units will meet the same quality standards.

The independently operated facilities are now challenging, and will continue to challenge the hospitals because surgeons in these facilities like the absence of red tape, simple record-keeping, close-in parking, compact corridors and operating areas.[1]

Moreover, the independently operated facilities result in lower charges, sometimes greater patient satisfaction, and potentially higher employee morale because of the small, close-knit nature of the enterprise. The owners of the facilities claim that patients receive a high degree of personal attention, which is not always the case in the nation's 7,000 hospitals.

Another advantage is that the patient's family is saved the inconvenience of visitor restrictions such as length of visit, number of visitors, poor parking facilities and long walks down distant corridors.

Since many hospitals' surgical facilities and beds are at capacity now, the community will benefit if "independents" fill this void.

To date the following views are held by various groups. The American Hospital Association (AHA) tends to favor short-stay surgery to be performed in general acute hospitals rather than in independently operated surgical facilities. However, the American Medical Association has a definite interest in independently operated ambulatory surgical centers, and tends to favor such programs over those controlled and operated within hospitals. To my knowledge, they have issued no official policy statement.

Although the federal government has not made a clear policy statement, it favors a system that will generate the lowest costs. The strongest evidence of this is the high likelihood that PSROs will generate an increase in the number of ambulatory surgical procedures that will take place in the U.S. in the near future. The federal Medicare program reimburses only *hospitals* for outpatient surgery, except through a few demonstration projects.

The Joint Commission on Accreditation of Hospitals (JCAH) has adopted guidelines that may soon become standards for ambulatory surgery. These guidelines hold that in order to minimize duplication of services, the objectives and plans of the ambulatory surgery center should be coordinated with those of other health service providers and planning agencies in the community. The main thrust of JCAH is on quality care, in sharp contrast to the policy advocated by the federal government and certain other sources which tend to emphasize cost. Efficiently run units both in hospitals and in independently operated facilities can fully meet the future requirements of the JCAH. Those hospitals that have an established short-stay surgical unit have found it generally to be a definite service to the community, to patients, and to physicians. Such units help the hospital to promote the establishment of a totally well-rounded program in terms of facilities available for patient care. To the extent that existing surgical facilities can be utilized to handle short-stay surgery, this has the further effect of increasing the utilization of ancillary departments, and, as a result, fixed costs of many areas of the hospital are spread over a larger number of units. Therefore, fiscal advantages can accrue in most situations by having a solid program of ambulatory surgery.

Hospitals that do not at the present time have an ambulatory surgery program are, in some cases, thoroughly investigating the concept. As noted by Michigan Blue Cross, "Hospitals are not running over each other to set up ambulatory surgical units. Their big reason is that they create no *new* health dollars by doing so; they only reallocate existing dollars."[2] In such hospitals and in communities in general where a surplus of hospital beds exists, the advent of ambulatory surgery could create financial problems if supported on a large scale. It is estimated that Massachusetts has twice the number of hospital beds it needs. According to James Latham, provider reimbursement manager for Blue Cross of Massachusetts, guided by an estimate, "The real savings will be in closing hospitals that don't have to be there."

Most physicians support the concept of ambulatory surgery. Drs. Wallace Reed and John Ford from the Phoenix Surgicenter® have been quoted as saying, "the future is almost unlimited; the surgical center can function successfully with greater savings to the patient while maintaining high standards of care, and such centers will be a necessity under national health insurance; the patient who comes to the hospital for minor surgery is subsidizing the ones who have major surgery.[3] While many physicians believe that ambulatory surgery should be performed in the independently operated facilities, others fully support the program in hospitals. The real challenge among hospitals is to provide convenience to the physician and the patient in order to compete economically with the advent of independently operated ambulatory surgical facilities. Some physicians express concern over malpractice issues in promoting ambulatory surgery.

Blue Cross has a general overriding concern regarding facilities for ambulatory surgery. The major conclusion of the organization is that such facilities should exist only when duplication is minimized. (See Chapter 22.) When a specific community has sufficient hospital facilities to provide care for meeting the needs of ambulatory surgery, independently operated facilities should be discouraged from being created, since their creation would tend to increase the community cost of medical care. If hospital facilities are insufficient, then freestanding independently operated programs could have a definite advantage for health care delivery within a specific community. Not all commercial insurance companies recognize outpatient surgery as a valid procedure for insurance coverage, hence, they "encourage" patients to be hospitalized rather than be discharged the same day.

MAJOR AREAS OF RESEARCH NECESSARY IN AMBULATORY SURGERY

A series of hypotheses are recommended for research consideration in the area of ambulatory surgery. Since they are hypotheses, they are not intended to constitute facts. Throughout much of the literature some of these statements, and similar statements, appear as conclusions. I would maintain, however, that many of these statements are made without the author having had any documented research data to back-up his statement(s).

Hypotheses

The purpose of this section is not to describe a theoretical framework or a research design that will specifically give the steps for testing these hypotheses. It is merely to identify some fruitful research areas that should be considered.

1. *An increase in supply (of ambulatory surgical facilities) tends to produce an increase in demand (incidence of) ambulatory surgical procedures.* Data is necessary to find out the situations and instances in which this statement might be true, and in which instances it would not be true, and why. It would be wrong for a community to assume that statements such as this are true without knowing the circumstances under which they might be factual or nonfactual.

2. *As a hospital develops and/or promotes an active ambulatory surgical program, it has a nondeleterious effect on total operating room activity, and, in fact, tends to increase the total number of surgical procedures performed.* Research into this area would indicate the impact upon hospitals in terms of operating room activity if short-stay surgery were promoted. For example, some may theorize that the ambulatory surgery patients would be the same patients that were now inpatients and that this would tend to have no effect on total operations performed. Many argue against this because new activity can be generated from physician and dental offices when hospitals open or enlarge ambulatory surgery facilities.

3. *Total hospital inpatient days are not affected by the development of an ambulatory short-stay surgery program if there is a high backlog of elective and urgent patients which tends to keep a hospital's occupancy level high.* If a low occupancy existed, under certain circumstances, occupancy could be reduced in those hospitals where ambulatory surgery is developed. Certainly in doing a study on this area, other issues would have to be examined, including the amount of new surgery that would be attracted from physician and dental offices. Another hypothesis would be: *Overall average length of stay varies inversely with the extent of ambulatory surgery performed.* (See Chapter 12, item six.)

4. *Under certain circumstances, with the establishment of a freestanding ambulatory center operated independently from the hospital, there would be no affect on inpatient days and number of OR procedures at a given hospital.* This is an important issue that would need to be resolved, and much data is needed before we can shed any light on the truth or falsehood of this statement.

5. *Surgery that is not medically necessary does not develop from the establishment of facilities to perform ambulatory surgery.* Some authors have claimed that the incidence of unneeded surgery has increased because of the advent of ambulatory surgical units, both inhospital and outside hospitals. There is no data to support this. Research is needed before such a conclusion could be given.

6. *The impact of hospitalization insurance programs on promoting or reducing the incidence of ambulatory surgery depends upon many factors.* Medicare insurance tends to reduce the incidence because at the present time it does not finance many nonhospital centers. Certain commercial insurances policies (other than Blue Cross) may provide coverage only when the patient is hospitalized. Many other factors need to be evaluated here.

7. *Hospital charges for ambulatory surgery exceed direct costs, and such excess income helps underwrite the complex operative procedures performed, such as kidney transplants.*

8. *One-third of all hospital operations could be performed on a same-day basis saving our nation's health care delivery system between $6 billion and $15 billion per year.*[4]

Notes

1. "Surgeons at freestanding centers say they are spared much hospital red tape and can retain the kind of independence they enjoy in private practice." Theodore Irwin, "We Need More Same Day Surgical Centers," *Today's Health,* January 1976, p. 10.

2. "In & Out Surgery," *Perspective,* Third Quarter, 1974, Blue Cross-Blue Shield of Michigan, p. 3.

3. *Ibid.,* p. 10.

4. "An Answer to Soaring Hospital Costs?" *Business Week,* July 7, 1976, p. 62.

Chapter 4
The Mechanics of Ambulatory Surgery

Thomas R. O'Donovan

The purpose of this chapter is to explore the specific details of ambulatory surgery and the dynamic cost implications. Included here will be how a facility can establish prices for care rendered, and what factors shall influence the prices charged. How does this pricing differ from inpatient pricing, role of "cost-based" pricing, and effect of competition on pricing? Do hospitals inflate ambulatory surgery prices to help finance expensive major surgery, such as kidney transplants? Should charges be itemized for each procedure, or would it be better to establish an all-inclusive rate? Should hospitals have different color-coded charge tickets for ambulatory surgery charge tickets?

One of the important decisions to be made early is whether or not the health care facility should establish a single price for each ambulatory surgery procedure or itemize each service performed for each procedure on the patient's bill.

Although hospitals, for the most part, cannot have different charges for the same tests or procedures for different patients because of Blue Cross and Medicare regulations, certain modifications can be made if they are cost justified. For example, if a hospital charges $200 for the first hour of surgery for a typical inpatient procedure, it may establish a price of $100 for an ambulatory procedure because it can be shown that most ambulatory procedures are shorter than many of the inpatient procedures.

More research is needed to determine whether or not it is justifiable to charge a different price for procedures that tend to be similar under both an inpatient and outpatient basis, such as a Dilation and Curettage (D&C). If a D&C is surgically the same in the operating room for the inpatient as it is for the ambulatory patient, can we justify a different price for the operation? We need more information before deciding whether or not a surgeon might say that the reason a particular patient has been hospitalized for one or two days rather then being treated as an outpatient is that the nature of the procedure is

27

different, e.g., that one D&C can be different from another. At the present time, there are no conclusive answers to these issues.

Itemization versus a single price structure tends to vary even among the freestanding, independently operated facilities. It should also be noted that the standard of practice tends to vary among different localities of the U.S., which can have a significant impact on charging systems. For example, in certain localities it is common practice for ambulatory surgical patients to receive a chest x-ray and an ECG. Such diagnostic precautions are not taken on many patients in the state of Michigan or in most other states. If we wanted to compare prices for services charged between one locale and another, we would have to know what the local practice is, because if certain required procedures and tests were performed on all patients in one locale, and on *no patients* in another locale, we would have no basis for comparison.

In addition, there is no day rate for a hospital bed for outpatient surgical procedures because there is no overnight confinement. Some may argue that part of the cost is still incurred, such as nursing, and for preop and postop care. Nevertheless, such services can be covered in the operating room charge.

Generally speaking, the freestanding independently operated units tend to establish a single charge for each ambulatory surgery procedure, rather than itemize all services rendered. Among hospitals, the practice varies widely. There is no way to document one system that is best. Some hospitals defend itemizing each service, and others defend the single blanket charge for a given procedure. The objective is to have the price match the service performed, so that patients are not treated differently. Another objective is to simplify billing procedures.

An issue to consider in regard to having an all-inclusive rate for ambulatory surgery patients, is that in many hospitals the accounting department needs the itemization approach because they are required to have the financial data that results from having separate charges for the completion of cost reports to third party payers.

If the breakdown of information were required from the accounting department because of Blue Cross or Medicare requirements in a particular hospital that used an all-inclusive rate approach, it would be necessary for their accounting department to "interpolate" the allocation of any future increases in charges. If a hospital charged the same for a kidney transplant as a hernia operation, there would be an outcry of inappropriateness because of the higher cost of the kidney transplant operation. Hospitals must be aware of allegations they they overprice certain services and procedures in order to help underwrite the costs incurred for other procedures. For example, we have often heard the public claim that hospitals charge too much for ambulatory surgical procedures to pay for the cost of the highly sophisticated procedures. This brings us to the issue of pricing of hospital services in all its ancillary departments, including room rates, EEG charges, x-ray procedures, laboratory tests, etc., to cover total costs, rather than establish certain ancillary charges with high profit margins that offset those areas that are operated at a loss. It should be noted that under the Medicare regulations, reimbursement is made at the lower of total costs *or* charges. This regulation is forcing hospitals to make absolutely certain that charges are set sufficiently high enough to insure that charges exceed costs.

The recommendation of this author is that hospitals should charge for each service separately. For each ambulatory surgical procedure performed, the patient should receive an itemized bill showing the individual charge of each item. If a hospital—for whatever reason—prefers an alternate system of a blanket price for each procedure, the approach could certainly be defended as equally sound as the recommended approach. Itemizing charges for both surgery and anesthesia requires a certain amount of cost analysis, both in establishing the original charge and in keeping it up-to-date. This, therefore, is one of the arguments in favor of a blanket charge. If charges are itemized, it would be appropriate to establish a surgery charge based on time spent on the procedure for the first half-hour and for increments of so much per half-hour thereafter. The same principle would apply in determining the anesthesia charge as well as the post anesthesia recovery (PAR) charge. If a medical anesthesiologist is performing the anesthesia, his billing will be separate, of course. Regardless of whether or not that is the case, the hospital can have an anesthesia charge based on time spent.

Another argument that is often advanced in favor of the blanket charging approach is that ambulatory procedures tend to be quite simple and do not need x-ray, CSR charges, or unusual pharmacy charges. Most hospitals itemize. The Phoenix Surgicenter® has a blanket charge, but the Ambulatory Surgical Facility of Hollywood, Florida itemizes.

The point of whether to itemize specific charges for services rendered or establish an all inclusive rate, in the end result, may not be relevant. It should be remembered that under today's system, most patients do not pay full charges but rather are insured through the major third parties (Blue Cross, Medicare and Medicaid) which pay the cost of rendering that care. As a result, little inequity results from the hospital pricing policies.

HOW TO DETERMINE PRICES

How should a facility establish prices for care rendered, and what factors should influence the prices charged? Prices should be based upon costs plus a reasonable mark-up. Independently operated facilities that are set up on a "for profit'' basis have to establish prices that will not only cover costs of depreciation, supplies, manpower, etc., but also to cover property taxes and profit for a return on the investment of the owners, (items that are not applicable in the "not for profit" hospital facility). This doesn't mean that the nonprofit hospital will not have prices that are far above costs. As previously discussed, it has often been alleged that hospitals charge higher prices than necessary for ambulatory surgical procedures in order to help pay for expensive procedures. Nevertheless, the basic principle applies: prices should reflect costs plus whatever mark-ups are necessary to reflect the nature of the enterprise.

Area practice is often an important factor in pricing, although in the health care industry it is much less a factor than in the automobile or steel industry. Our research revealed that area practice for ambulatory surgery pricing in hospitals varied widely across the nation. The methods used to establish the prices (such as blanket versus itemization) also varied. There is certainly no collusion among hospitals to fix prices.

Health care facilities should increase their prices whenever they are cost justified. The typical approach is for cost increase projections to be made for the following budget period and a schedule of price increases (either at the beginning or during the budget period) to be established by financial personnel. Modifications can be made when experience occurs that is different from the assumptions made. A sound approach to budgeting is essential in any and all instances. In the chapters presented in Parts II and III there are several case studies illustrating specific issues and examples in pricing.

Role of Coded Charge Tickets

Should color-coded charge tickets be established for separating ambulatory surgery charges from regular inpatient charges? This approach is commonly performed in hospitals where there is a separate facility for ambulatory surgery (such as at Santa Barbara Cottage Hospital). In hospitals where the ambulatory surgery is merged with the regular inpatient surgery, this approach can still be taken. In a hospital such as Mount Carmel Mercy Hospital, where a computer system prices all charge tickets, it is less necessary to identify charge tickets separately. It is an individual situation for each hospital.

WHEN SHOULD LAB WORK BE DONE

Should patients be required to report a day or so before their ambulatory surgery procedure for lab work, or can the necessary lab work be done on the morning of surgery? This is another practice that varies considerably. The more convenient ambulatory surgery is for physicians and patients, the more likely it will be practiced. The independently operated facilities have the capability for this routine lab work, and in most cases, the patients have such work performed on the morning of surgery. In hospitals it is interesting to note the various approaches taken. In some hospitals the bureaucratic structure interferes with getting the blood drawn, tests performed, and results on the morning of surgery. Most hospitals strongly prefer having the blood work done approximately one or two days before surgery so that the information is available when the procedure begins.

A few years ago when Mt. Carmel Mercy Hospital embarked on its program of ambulatory surgery, the chief of surgery strongly recommended that we make ambulatory surgery as convenient as possible by having the blood work done on the morning of surgery. This created a challenge because the lab was not set up to do it without a good deal of coordination efforts. (See Appendix H.) At a national conference of the American Academy of Medical Administrators in March 1973, ambulatory surgery was discussed. Those representing hospital programs tended to favor having the blood work done prior to the day of surgery. Every effort should be made to make health care delivery efficient and convenient for physicians, patients, etc. If, therefore, the hospital can, without undue costs and complications, perform these procedures on the morning of surgery, it should do so. On the other hand, if doing so creates problems, then the patient should report for blood work prior to the day of surgery.

STEPS IN SETTING UP A PROGRAM

How does a hospital go about establishing a sound program of ambulatory surgery? The answer is "very carefully." We examined this issue in a large number of hospitals that were able to establish a successful program of ambulatory surgery. In virtually every case a committee of some kind had been formed in order to launch the project. Initial support must come from either the administration of the hospital, the board of trustees, or the medical staff, though the motivation can come from more than one source. In any event, hospital administrators should insure that the process is properly managed and that input is obtained from all key areas.

If a committee is charged with the objective of examining the implications of ambulatory surgery with a possible view to establishing a program, it is extremely important to have medical staff representation (particularly anesthesiology, general surgery, and gyn surgery). Of course, plastic surgery and many other surgical subspecialties will eventually be interested in the program, but their membership on the original committee, while valuable, is not necessarily crucial. Other representation should include administration, nursing, and perhaps someone from the office of the controller. Administrative representatives in different facilities have varying degrees of effectiveness. In some hospitals one of the early objectives is an evaluation of whether or not an ambulatory surgery program *should* be created. At other hospitals *that* objective will be assumed, and the approach will be what *steps* should be taken to create such a program. Every effort should be made to avoid having the issue become a political football within the medical staff. Hospitals have enough problems with political issues without deliberately attempting to create another one. Ambulatory surgery should be a perfect example of a "safe" issue that can see a great deal of cooperation between the staff, administration, and other elements of the hospital.

Once a firm decision has been made to establish an ambulatory surgery program major issues need to be resolved. A subcommittee can be formed to handle the construction and financial details, such as costs, and location of the unit (creating a separate tailormade unit or merging it within the existing inpatient system). The physicians will concentrate on the professional aspects. Without the support of the surgeons, the program will die an early death. Anesthesia is a key issue too, because many ambulatory surgery programs have not been able to do an effective job because of the absence of a sufficient number of anesthesiologists. It is not useful to list a number of *specific* steps that a hospital should take in order to establish a program of ambulatory surgery. Each situation is different, and approaches must reflect local needs.

After a hospital has a solid program of ambulatory surgery, there will still be occasional situations of *rejection* by certain members of the medical staff. One case is recalled of a large hospital with an active ambulatory surgery program. One of the physicians involved in the direction of the unit was very pleased one day when a high-status surgeon admitted a young adult to the program for a hernia. Up to that time this surgeon had never once utilized the ambulatory surgery program of the hospital. A few weeks later these two physicians were discussing it in the hallway, and the surgeon who had handled the case mentioned that he never realized what an excellent approach to medical care this was until he had actually experienced it first-hand. The doctor was elated because he knew that by *this* surgeon using the facility, other "slow movers" would also. In effect, the surgeon was being a catalyst which would tend to stimulate other surgeons to use the unit.

Barriers To Overcome

It is important to note how some of the restraints on ambulatory surgery tie in with the inpatient approach. We know that there is a great deal of pressure from the government and Blue Cross to reduce the length of stay. Some of the obstacles involve inpatient activity as well as ambulatory surgery. For example, a physician before discharging a patient needs to know that follow-up care will be adequate so that the prognosis of the patient will not be endangered. If an OB patient is in the hospital to deliver her eighth child and she has no help at home, the physician might be more likely to discharge her after six days than after three days. In other words, the physician considers the home environment as part of the medical care. If a patient is supposed to go to a nursing home after his hospitalization and the family is having difficulty finding an acceptable facility, there may be one or more days of delay in discharge because of the "mechanics" of the nursing home placement. Home care can only be effective when there is some form of help for the patient at home in addition to the medical personnel that will visit him.

How many times have we seen physicians discharge a patient on the weekend because the family insisted that no one was available to drive the patient home on Thursday or Friday. In fact, it would be interesting to note the percentages of total discharges for each day of the week, throughout America. Similarly, if the home situation isn't conducive to recovery, the physician may be quite reluctant to utilize ambulatory surgery for a particular patient.

Hospitals are also concerned about credit policies. Since ambulatory surgeries are generally elective procedures, controllers like to have payment assured before the surgery takes place. The same is often true for inpatient elective surgery. The patient's insurance policy information is obtained by the hospital from the patient after the doctor's office "books" the patient. Deposits are usually required if insurance is missing or is in any way inadequate.

To promote financial stability, many hospitals require a 3 to 6 day notice before an ambulatory surgery patient can be operated on. This gives the business office time to verify that financial details are intact. But many doctors may want to book some patients sooner if the operating room time is available. This can serve to limit the utilization of ambulatory surgery, but can be corrected by a compromise. In most cases two days is enough time for the business office to garner credit information, and both the patient and the surgeon are better served by the availability of reduced waiting time for elective ambulatory surgery.

COST IMPLICATIONS OF AMBULATORY SURGERY

One of the serious shortcomings of the literature on ambulatory surgery is the set of conclusions relating to cost that have no factual documentation. It is commonly stated that ambulatory surgery reduces costs, although it is unclear if cost is defined as community cost, facility cost, or merely charges paid by an insurance company. Much research is necessary in cost determination before definitive answers can be established.

Under some circumstances ambulatory surgery can *increase* both total costs and unit costs. If a hospital is operating at 80% occupancy and if it embarks upon an ambitious ambulatory surgery program the occupancy may be reduced to 75%. If there is no reduction in the number of personnel commensurate with the reduction in inpatients, an increase in unit cost could result. In this instance, many fiscal challenges would also begin to arise. The issue of costs versus billings further complicates the issue.

In another instance, say a hospital builds a unit for the sole purpose of ambulatory surgery, creating a certain level of staffing. If the number of operations performed is much lower than estimated, it could become a losing venture, increasing health care costs both for the community as well as for the hospital. Nevertheless, it is true that a proper level of ambulatory surgery can reduce long-run health care delivery costs in the U.S. or in any country.

Analysis of these concepts reveals the complexity of the issue. If, for example, a hospital with a high backlog of elective and urgent cases, institutes an ambulatory surgery program, the average length of stay tends to increase because the short-stay procedures are being eliminated. In this case, the total costs incurred by the facility will increase. At the same time, the community may be better served because more patients are being cared for while the backlog of elective surgery is being reduced by ambulatory surgery. The long-range advantage might be a decrease in future construction of inpatient beds in the immediate community served by that particular hospital. Throughout our history, when large backlogs of elective surgery existed, there was a great deal of pressure for the construction of additional beds. Active programs of ambulatory surgery can certainly reduce the need for future bed construction. The complexity arises in determining whether or not the backlog is growing or static. If the hospital had a static backlog and embarked upon an ambitious program of ambulatory surgery, eliminating the backlog, the potential effect might be poor utilization. Specifically, if the need for beds eased up, the physicians might feel less pressure to discharge patients than they would if there was a huge backlog of elective surgery. The same thing could apply in the Department of Internal Medicine, etc., in regard to bed utilization.

Unless a proper approach is taken to the cost issue, the result can be many erroneous conclusions. Some of the data collected on ambulatory surgery—unless properly interpreted—will not tell us whether, in a given hospital, we are *reducing* costs or *shifting* costs. This is the problem of community costs versus the individual hospital's costs, as we have described.

In 1975 Mount Carmel Mercy Hospital performed 1,246 ambulatory surgery procedures. We do not have specific information on whether or not these procedures were done on patients who would have been *inpatients* for one to three days at Mount Carmel, or at another hospital, or whether or not these procedures were shifted from other hospitals, doctors' offices, the emergency department, or the outpatient department. Knowledge of that kind of information is essential in order to draw sound conclusions. We are, therefore, unable to say whether or not the 1,246 ambulatory surgical procedures at Mount Carmel in 1975 reduced health care costs for the community, for the hospital, for both, or for neither. In the short run, the cost impact would be minimal, but in the long run, a substantial reduction in community cost is possible.

According to the American Hospital Association, in 1974 the total number of operations in U.S. hospitals was 16,839,217. One approach to measure the impact of ambulatory surgery on cost savings is to compare the number of operations performed on an ambulatory basis with the number that *should* have been performed on an ambulatory basis. Much of the literature suggests a range of 20 to 40%, so we will use 30%. In any given hospital or locality, that figure will depend on the type of hospital, the amount and quality of anesthesia available, the current number of procedures, insurance implications, and patient and physician acceptance. The literature suggests that if a hospital converts a proper amount of its inpatient surgery to outpatient surgery, over one-half of the hospital bill would be eliminated. (See Table 4:1.) This assumption requires further research. We could determine the amount of hospital cost savings throughout the United States by determining the cost savings using the assumption previously described.

Applying that model to Hospital X in Table 4:1, we find that if 11,000 operations were performed in a given year, and if 1,000 of them were done on an ambulatory basis (assuming 30% of the total could have been performed on an ambulatory basis) we subtract 1,000 from 30% of 11,000 or 3,300 minus 1,000 which equals 2,300. If the difference in charge between an inpatient stay and the same procedure performed on an ambulatory basis were $270, then multiplying $270 times 2,300 shows that this hospital could save $621,000 per year by a complete ambulatory surgery program.[1] The finding however, is false. While *billings* would be reduced by $621,000, it would not decrease total costs by $621,000 per year because many hospitals are "cost reimbursed" for most of their activity. This is especially true if the hospital superimposed their ambulatory surgery program upon their existing inpatient program. If, for example, the hospital added no nurses, constructed no operating rooms, or incurred no interest or depreciation expense increases, the only major increase in cost associated with these 1,000 cases would be supply costs. Therefore, upon further examination, it is extremely difficult to determine the actual cost saving at this hospital or in the community with a complete ambulatory surgery program.

Under certain assumptions, the hospital in Table 4:1 for a given year could charge $163 for a typical ambulatory surgery case, and perform 1,100 in that

TABLE 4:1   PRICE COMPARISONS OF DILATION AND CURETTAGES (D&Cs)

Service	Hospital 2-Day In-Patient Stay ($)	Hospital Ambulatory Surgery Basis($)
Room rate	194	-0-
Operating room charge	200	95
Anesthesia (non-MD)*	(100)	(40)
Anesthesia (MDA); (hospital charge)	60	20
IV therapy	9	9
Pharmacy	7	-0-
PAR	35	25
CSR-Medical, surgical supplies	7	-0-
X-ray	-0-	-0-
Admission kit	4	-0-
Lab (required tests)		
CBC	9	9
VDRL	5	-0-
SMA 12	18	-0-
Urinalysis	5	5
SMA 6	15	-0-
Average of additional lab charges	50	-0-
TOTAL	$618	$163

*Most ambulatory surgery patients are attended to by an MDA, and therefore the $100 and $40 figures do not appear in the totals.

NOTE: The prices were taken from a hospital in the Midwestern United States, 1976.

given year, generating $179,300 in billings, a $36,333 increase in revenue, and an $11,000 increase in costs.[2] Such startling results could not occur in an independently operated facility under the U.S. system of cost-reimbursed hospital care. These assumptions are:

1. Hospital does 40% Blue Cross business on a system of cost plus 2%; 45% Medicare and Medicaid at cost; and 15% commercial insurance and "direct pay." It should be noted that the Michigan Blue Cross plan is only one of a very few plans that maintain the 2% add-on factor. Other plans pay on a variety of methods including cost, charges, negotiated rate, and prospective rate.

2. Hospital performs the 1,100 surgical procedures without constructing new operating rooms, hiring additional nurses and/or admitting clerks; and the increase in costs incurred as a result of the 1,100 procedures were lab reagents and surgical supplies amounting to an average of $10 per patient. (One might question this assumption, because if 1,100 surgical procedures are performed out of 11,000 total for a given hospital, it might often be necessary to employ at least one additional nurse. If it

wasn't necessary, it would indicate that the hospital was originally over-staffed.)
3. Patients cared for followed the same mix as in "1" above.

Ignoring such issues as role of bad debts, and cost allocations among inpatients and outpatients, the following calculations are made:
1. An average charge of $163 times 1,100 procedures equals $179,300 in billings.
2. The revenue increase was $36,333, which was determined by ascertaining the cost increase for "cost-reimbursed" patients and increase in billings for commercial insurance patients and "direct pays."
   a) Blue Cross; 40% of 1,100 times $10 plus 2% = 440 times $10 plus $88 = $4,488.
   b) Medicare-Medicaid; 45% of 1,100 times $10 = $4,950.
   c) Commercial insurance and direct pay patients; 15% of 1,100 times $163 = $26,895.
3. The $10 described in assumption "b" is only a "short-run incremental cost" which would not hold true in the intermediate or long-run except under the most unusual circumstances. The $10 is not a "true-cost" and would never appear, as such, in official hospital year-end financial reports.

What happens if you change the assumptions? The major conclusions of this analysis would not change because reimbursement systems are not completely different in all parts of the country. The conclusions also do not change in those states with prior rate review in effect, or in hospitals operating under prospective reimbursement. In Florida, Blue Cross is not "cost plus 2%"; the hospitals are reimbursed charges for Blue Cross patients, generally, but Medicare percentages are *much* higher than the 45% used in our example. Though all the numerical assumptions are different in Florida, the bottom line still comes out the same. Whenever assumption "2" holds true, the cost reimbursement system of hospital care in America results in a greater community cost when independently operated surgical facilities are erected.

The heart of the cost issue in "hospitals versus the independents" lies in the assumptions made. If we assume that our health care delivery system is—or should be—operating under a free enterprise system (private practice plus open market capitalism in its complete form where price truly influences "quantity produced," etc.), the lower prices charged by the independently operated ambulatory surgical facility would reduce community health care costs.[3]

But these assumptions are nowhere close to being true. They might be desirable, but they are not facts. Health care operates far more like public utilities. The uniqueness of health care is the cost-reimbursement feature wherein well over one-half of all hospital revenue comes from costs incurred, not prices charged. No other major industry in America has such a system. This, then, is the major reason for the dilemma in resolving the issue of whether or not hospital ambulatory surgery is less costly to the community than the same surgery performed in independently operated facilities.

A MACROVIEW

Under what assumptions could the creation of independently operated facilities reduce community health care costs? Over a period of a few years, community costs of health care would decrease when:

- A community need for ambulatory surgery facilities exists.
- Present health care facilities are operating at capacity.
- An avoidance of some construction of additional hospital facilities occurs.
- The charges for ambulatory surgery procedures of the newly created independently operated facility (or facilities) are less than what would be received in reimbursement by the hospital (or hospitals) if that hospital (or hospitals) were created.
- Other factors influencing this community cost reduction would be the closing of certain outmoded hospital facilities and not replacing them (either in full or in part) because one or more independent surgical facilities filled the gap adequately; also, if the "cost reimbursement" feature in hospital health care delivery were eliminated, then, depending on the new system that would replace it, this could result in a decrease in community costs.

Applying this model on a national basis, we assume that of the 17 million operations performed in the U.S. in a given year, 4%[4] were done on an ambulatory basis. If the proper level should be 30%, we take 30% of 17 million, or 5,100,000 and subtract the 4%, which gives us 68,000. This means that we are doing 5,032,000 too few ambulatory surgeries per year. If the typical savings on these procedures were $270 each, the annual savings to the U.S. is $1.4 billion. However, this does not include the role of the independently operated freestanding units or their affect on the $1.2 billion savings. Based upon the potential inadequacy of the assumptions and the lack of data in general, we venture to suggest that the $1.4 billion does not reflect a realistic total (it might be higher or lower).

In *Business Week* the case of a typical Chicago hospital which charged $480. for a particular operation was compared with Surgicare, the freestanding center in Chicago which charged only $169.[5] The implication was that the cost of the freestanding facility to the community was $311 lower than that of the hospital. The issue of true "costs" versus "billings" must be resolved. The magazine further suggested that a complete approach to ambulatory surgery in the U.S.

would reduce our health care expenditures by $6 billion to $15 billion per year. We believe, however, that more research is needed to evaluate these figures.

Let us examine Table 4:1 in detail. An effort was made to gather such information from several hospitals to determine if any common approach was taken. Such was not the case. Almost every hospital has its own unique approach to determining prices for ambulatory surgery. One of these areas that *was common* to most hospitals was the individual pricing of factors that make up ambulatory surgery, rather than a blanket charge for the overall procedure. Prices tend to change for the services listed in Table 4:1 every six to twelve months, due to inflationary factors.

Table 4:1 further describes the difference between the common charges for a two-day inpatient stay for a D&C versus the same procedure done on an ambulatory surgery basis. Prices would vary for those D&C procedures when the patient was in the hospital *one* day, or *three or more* days. It would be uncommon, however, for a D&C patient to stay in the hospital for more than two days unless there was a secondary diagnosis. In fact, some physicians claim there is even a difference between most two-day D&Cs compared with those done on an ambulatory basis. Older patients, or those for whom certain complications are expected, would more likely be hospitalized for the procedure. We must conclude that there can be a difference between an inpatient D&C and an outpatient D&C even though the diagnosis is the same.

Similarily, there can be differences in any procedure. One obvious example is a hernia in a 50-year-old adult compared with one in a young child. It is difficult to take a mass statistical approach in drawing conclusions about differential patterns of extending patient care. Nevertheless, there are enough similarities between D&Cs throughout the nation to find the approach taken in Table 4:1 to be useful.

Table 4:1 shows that the inpatient charge for two days in a semi-private room is $97 per day, compared to a zero charge for ambulatory surgery. Some might argue that there are some costs in ambulatory surgery relative to the room in terms of a minimum amount of nursing care and the use of a cot as noted earlier in this chapter. Some hospitals charge a nominal amount of $25 or $50 to include such costs. The operating room charge of $200 is a charge based on the first hour, and this particular hospital charges $50 per half-hour for each additional half-hour in the operating room. Since it is rare for a D&C to go beyond an hour, we have entered $200 as the charge for the inpatient stay. This hospital has a policy of charging for ambulatory surgery at the rate of $95 for the first half-hour, and $50 for each additional half-hour. There are some ambulatory surgery procedures that may take 35 or 45 minutes, and the charge for the operating room for those procedures would be $95 plus $50, or $145. Table 4:1 assumes that the operation would take less than a half-hour.

If a hospital has nurse anesthetists available, as well as anesthesiologists, there may be a higher charge when a nurse anesthetist assists. At this hospital the charge is $100 for the first hour when a nurse anesthetist is present; the price schedule goes up from there to reflect additional time elements. The same is true in ambulatory surgery. In totalling the two columns, we have used the anesthesiologist approach because it is typical in this particular hospital. When the anesthesiologist performs the case, the charge is $60 for the hospital charge for an inpatient (based on time), and $20 for ambulatory surgery (based on time). In most cases, patients are given an IV for which there is a $9 charge both to inpatients and outpatients. If the physician does not order an IV, there is no charge.

There is no specific pharmacy charge in either approach, but in examining the actual bills we find that there is an average pharmacy charge of $7 for a two-day inpatient D&C compared to *no pharmacy charges* on ambulatory patients.

The post anesthesia recovery room (PAR) has a charge of $35 for all inpatients, based on time, and $25 for ambulatory surgery patients. Some of the major inpatient cases incur a charge far above $35, but these are the minimum charges for minor procedures, such as D&Cs.

The medical-surgical supplies usually amount to about $7 per patient in the *inpatient* example, but they are rarely used for the ambulatory patient.

In the typical case, no x-ray procedures are done for D&C inpatients or outpatients.

The inpatients receive an inpatient kit, and a charge of $4 is added to their bill. Obviously, this does not apply to ambulatory patients, since they are not admitted.

Only two laboratory tests, totalling $14, are required at this hospital for ambulatory surgery patients. There are five required tests for all inpatients. In examining a large number of actual bills rendered for two-day D&C procedures, we found that the average bill showed an additional $50 in laboratory charges, whereas there were no additional charges for the D&C ambulatory patient.

The total charge averaged $618 for the two-day stay D&C inpatient, compared to only $163 for the ambulatory surgery D&C. We should not conclude that all of these D&Cs should have been done on an ambulatory basis. We cited extenuating circumstances in which the GYN physician feels that hospitalization is necessary because of the patient's condition. Nevertheless, since over 85% of all D&Cs performed at this hospital and many other hospitals are on an inpatient basis, we can safely say that a large percentage definitely could be done on an ambulatory basis were it not for the mitigating factors that have been described in Chapter 2.

OTHER COST ISSUES

There are many physicians across the country that automatically hospitalize all D&Cs. Others quite commonly utilize the ambulatory surgery department of the hospital for almost all of their D&C procedures. Likewise, some hospitals in the U.S. have a policy that all T&A patients must stay overnight for observation rather than be discharged on the day of surgery. At the Phoenix Surgicenter® and many of the independently operated surgical centers throughout the U.S., thousands of T&As are performed on an ambulatory basis. Can we say that the medical staff that establishes a policy of overnight stays is wrong? What determines the standard of care in a given locality? Is there any more danger of bleeding in a patient operated on at Hospital X in Connecticut versus Hospital Y in Arizona? Will PSROs establish norms of practice as to when certain procedures will result in requiring a patient to be discharged on the day of surgery versus a later date?

John Dillon, M.D., when giving his keynote address at the first national conference on ambulatory surgery sponsored by the American Academy of Medical Administrators, mentioned that, at UCLA Medical Center, none of the T&As are allowed to go home on the day of surgery. They must stay a minimum of one night in order to be observed for potential bleeding. He spent much time describing the rationale behind this.

We mentioned previously that many hospitals have differing schemes in regard to ambulatory surgery pricing. There are some hospitals that itemize all charges other than the use of the operating room, but instead of charging for the operating room based on time, they put a price for the use of the operating room on each procedure. Therefore, if any particular procedure takes a longer or shorter time than expected, the price remains the same, since the charge is determined ahead of time. Some have a charge for the first quarter-hour and for each quarter-hour thereafter of operating room use. Some hospitals have a different charge when local anesthesia is used rather than general anesthesia. There are many hospitals that have the same rates for outpatient surgery as well as inpatient surgery, the only difference being the room rate. Some hospitals charge a full day's room rate even though the patient may be in the hospital only three hours before being discharged. There are several other charging schemes utilized.

In summary, we can conclude that ambulatory surgery can result in long-run community health care cost reductions; in the short-run and intermediate-run, under certain conditions, ambulatory surgery could increase or decrease community health care costs, and an individual hospital's total cost. A large number of variables pull and tug in determining costs, and unless all the assumptions are spelled out carefully, conclusions should only be offered tentatively.

Gregg W. Downey[6] did a fine job in developing a model similar to this in his article on "A Scanner for Every Hospital?" He described the alleged impact of scanners on total hospital costs. He summarized the findings of an article that appeared in the October 1975 issue of *Radiology*. Drs. Wortzman, Holgate and Morgan reported on the cost savings of using the CT scanner by comparing certain studies, such as angiographic procedures, and pneumoencephalograms in which the use of the scanner was able to eliminate a certain number of hospital days. By taking the per diem rate per hospital inpatient day and multiplying the number of days saved, they showed an annual savings of $2,232,500. Since the scans cost $100 apiece, the total net savings is $2 million. Downey then says, "Skeptics, such as HEW's Rubel, are not especially impressed. 'You can do a lot with figures; is the scanner really saving money? Have they closed down their angiography? Did they actually get rid of their old equipment and reduce staffing? Was there any actual reduction of costs within the institution?' " In a word, no. The physicians acknowledged this at the conclusion of their article. " 'In terms of the global costs of medical care, the net figures given above could be misleading. If one does not close a hospital ward due to the shortened hospital stay and avoidance of admissions, the largest portion of the savings listed above would not be realized. In addition, a hospital administrator will point out that the per diem rate rises as the hospital stay is shortened and efficiency increases. Leaving one or five hospital beds empty does little to reduce hospital costs. A ward must be closed with the attendant reduction in hospital staff and, in spite of this, the per diem rate will still not drop in proportion to the percentage of beds closed because of certain fixed, irreducible costs. The savings listed above, however, indicate that CT would allow a more efficient use of the health care dollar, with hospital beds not taken up by patients with dementia, problem headaches, or epilepsy.' "

ROLE OF INCREMENTAL COSTS

One of the arguments used by prospective freestanding independently operated facilities in obtaining community support for construction is that the charges they will make for their procedures will be less than that currently charged by existing hospitals in the community. In fact, we have reviewed several staff reports prepared by health planning agencies, obtaining the following information: the proposed freestanding center would present its charges for typical operations to be performed, which would be compared with the charges made by local hospitals for the same procedures done on an ambulatory basis, and for inpatients staying for one or two days. In most cases the charges from the freestanding center were lower. The conclusion often drawn from such an analysis is that the cost to the community is lower when a freestanding unit performs ambulatory surgical procedures, rather than when a hospital does them.

There is an alternative way to approach this in order to determine the cost to the community. For example, if in all of the cases studied we assume that the hospitals were reimbursed primarily on the basis of costs incurred rather than charges, it would be important to calculate the incremental cost of a hospital providing those services versus not providing them. For example, if Hospital X in a certain community were performing 1,000 ambulatory surgical procedures a year in a unit that was merged with its inpatient activity (rather than a separate unit, as is the case of Santa Barbara Cottage Hospital in Santa Barbara, California), we would find that the costs of either eliminating the 1,000 procedures per year, or the incremental cost in adding 1,000 procedures per year divided by the per procedure charge made would show an entirely different figure. The only point is that comparing the prices of the hospital ambulatory surgical procedure with that of a proposed or existing freestanding facility is not the best way to determine the cost *to the community*. A much more sophisticated approach must be found. The concept of "incremental cost" is extremely important.

It should be noted, however, that true savings cannot be measured by merely comparing the charge of an operation in a hospital versus a free standing center. As a matter of fact, the basic charge for such a service is almost irrelevant because most patients do not pay the full charge. What must be done to determine the true cost savings is to compare the per unit *cost* of the surgery performed in a freestanding facility with what the *incremental per unit costs* would be if that total amount of surgery had been performed in the hospital. Based upon previously made statements in this chapter, it is believed that the facts would show that it could be less costly to the community to have an ambulatory surgery center located in the hospital. Although it is certain that ambulatory surgery will reduce our total national health care expenditures, we must be careful to fully examine this issue of costs before creating freestanding centers which create additional fixed costs. This argument can be challenged by the following: what if a hospital does not have a large percentage of its activity cost reimbursed?; and what about the direct pay patient who can go to one facility or the other and would stand to gain from lower prices in the non-hospital unit?

Medicare is cost reimbursed among our nation's hospitals, and Blue Cross varies from state to state.[7] Under prospective reimbursement, further challenges exist that complicate the issue; National Health Insurance, for example, may bring a whole new reimbursement scheme upon us.

The overall relationship of health care costs, charges, billings, and revenues is further complicated by the fact that over 90 percent of hospitals' billings are eventually collected after year-end cost settlements with third party payers.

Thus, there could be an argument advanced that both hospitals and independently operated facilities receive their total revenues based on prices charged.

ROLE OF AREA-WIDE PLANNING

The subject of health care costs in relation to ambulatory surgery has bounded around like a football throughout the press and in the literature on ambulatory surgery. Many assumptions are made, some of which may be valid and some may not, depending upon whether or not documented evidence can be obtained to test such assumptions.

For example, in Hartford, Connecticut a freestanding ambulatory surgery center applied for approval from local health planning officials.[8] A great deal of back-and-forth discussion occurred as a result of the proposal that was offered. An editorial appearing in the *Hartford Times,* a local newspaper, on January 7, 1976, reported a major story on how Connecticut's first ambulatory surgery center was approved. Many assumptions regarding costs were presented in the editorial. The following excerpts appeared:

"Commission member, Elizabeth Cathles, said she was concerned that the surgical center would have the effect of raising hospital rates. 'Hospitals are inevitably going to raise their rates if you take their low-cost items away from them,' she said. 'It may be unreasonable to expect that health care costs will be lowered by this outpatient surgery.' " She also expressed a concern about what she said were eleven unused surgery rooms at the three nearby hospitals. State Health Commissioner Douglas S. Lloyd, another Commission member, agreed with Mrs. Cathles. "The larger question is the unused surgical facilities now in existence. If we put more facilities in, the additional cost will be passed on, if not directly to the patient, then to the insurance companies. I'm not convinced there is a need for more surgical rooms when there are already facilities in the city not being used." Another Commission member suggested that the proposal should be approved if for no other reason than to teach the hospitals that the work can be done more economically at alternative health care facilities.

In the *Hartford Times* on the following day, January 8, 1976, there was a specific editorial regarding this issue. This editorial strongly supported having a freestanding ambulatory surgery facility separate from the hospital because of the impact it would have on the cost of delivery of health care in Hartford. "The state's hospitals stand to lose lucrative surgical business to the private Hartford Surgical Center, since the Center has proven indisputably that its rates will be lower than the rates presently charged by the hospitals."

There is no question that the newspaper heartily endorsed and actively supported the issuance of a license for the Hartford Surgical Center. A careful analysis of similar centers in other states clearly indicated a substantial savings for ambulatory surgical patients who avail themselves of the services of the private facilities instead of hospitals. An analysis of the Connecticut situation allegedly revealed that area hospitals use same-day surgical charges to supplement losses from other unprofitable activities, and that some area hospitals have unreasonable delays in scheduling ambulatory, nonemergency surgery, which results in psychological hardship and inconvenience to patients. The editorial stated that certain members of the Commission that opposed the provisional licensure will have an opportunity in the coming three years to examine the results of their vote. It concluded by saying that "in the meantime, Connecticut's ambulatory surgery patients will be saving thousands of dollars, as will the insurance companies which pay most of the bills."

This kind of editorial has appeared often in the United States, and while it contains a certain amount of truth, there is much to be done in relation to whether or not freestanding nonhospital units can really save health care dollars for a particular community or whether or not such surgery can be performed at a lower *total* cost by having existing hospital health care delivery systems perform this community service.

Hospitals that believe independently operated ambulatory surgery centers should not be allowed to exist should realize that the overall situation must be carefully probed, because the freestanding centers have a position that is loud and clear. Before hospitals reject their position, they should fully understand it.

Many such centers and physicians, both surgeons and anesthesiologists, have found excessive bureaucratic red tape to be quite a detriment to the delivery of sound health care in the area of ambulatory surgery. It is unfair to automatically choose one form or another without looking at the total gestalt.

Notes

1. The figure $270 is cited in some papers; but in the July 7, 1975 issue of *Business Week*, a figure of $311 is mentioned. At Hospital X an estimate for a D&C differential was calculated to $455 as noted in Table 4:1. In this example we used the conservative figure of $270. Hospitals with low occupancy (less than 80%) which embark on an ambitious program of ambulatory surgery will not only have to be concerned with a possible further reduction in occupancy, but also with their pricing system; the pricing model in Table 4:1 may result in comparison with inpatient charges.

2. The figure of $36,333 does not include the surgeons' anesthesiologists' fees.

3. Theodore Irwin, "We Need More Same-Day Surgical Centers," *Today's Health*, January 1976, p. 52. Because of the volume of patients treated, the Phoenix Surgicenter® estimates it saved patients more than $1 million and more than 17,000 days that would have been spent in a hospital. It also saved about $4 million in construction costs for additional hospital facilities.

4. The 4% figure is merely an estimate.

5. *Business Week*, July 7, 1975, p. 62. (Reprinted as Appendix H).

6. *Modern Healthcare,* February 1976, p. 16s-16w.

7. New York Blue Cross tends to thwart ambulatory surgery since it reimburses such procedures on an outpatient basis similar to emergency department charging, and, therefore, hospitals can get better reimbursement if the patient is held overnight as an inpatient.

8. See Appendix A.

Chapter 5
Major Issues of Construction and Design

Barbara Bregande

It is conceivable that a hospital could maintain one to three same-day surgical programs as census and service area dictates, e.g., an outpatient clinic type same-day olram-department, use of the hospital OR-service, and the building of a remotely located satellite for same-day surgery. Same-day surgical programs are geared to procedures that generally require a properly controlled environment commonly found in the hospital's operating room suite, but not exclusively with those procedures requiring the use of inhalation anesthetics.

Hospitals with busy outpatient and emergency departments will probably continue to perform same-day surgery whether or not a more formal service is developed. However, some of the procedures commonly performed in these departments might be performed better in a same-day service or department because scheduling, staff skills, and the aseptic environment can be controlled more effectively. Many of these so-called outpatient procedures often fall into the gray area of cases which could be treated in an operating room suite, a freestanding facility, *or* a physician's office. They are called shifting procedures. Presently, they include oral surgical procedures, dental, plastic and radiological procedures, and almost all "scopics." Most can be performed under local or inhalation anesthesia, in a sterile or nonsterile environment, on a same-day or short-stay basis, or in a physician's office. Where these procedures are performed depends on the following: (1) size of the hospital; (2) skill of the surgeon; (3) surgical technique; and (4) the mental and physical condition of the patient.

Determining which shifting procedures should be performed in an operating room environment appears to be a major obstacle in planning same-day surgical programs and facilities. The major question is whether or not office procedures belong in a same-day surgical service, and if third-party payers should provide facility reimbursement.

Surgeons perform shifting procedures in the office in the following situations: when the procedure will not be painful for the patient or cause undue

47

anxiety; when the patient's physical condition places him in a low risk category; when local or inhalation anesthesia will be used for a very short duration
and will provide the desired degree of relaxation; and when surgical judgment
dictates that the procedure will be an entity unto itself, i.e., without the need or
possibility of secondary surgical intervention. A negative response to any of
these factors can cause the surgeon to decide to perform the procedure in an
operating room or other type hospital environment. The responsibility for
choosing the proper location for a given patient procedure rests entirely on the
attending surgeon. Since some office procedures belong in the operating room
environment, they should be reimbursable from third-party payors.

HOW A HOSPITAL IDENTIFIES ITS POTENTIAL CASELOAD

Some authorities believe that 20-40% of a hospital's operating room
caseload constitutes the type of surgery that can be performed on a same-day
basis. The Innovative Programs, Incorporated, (IPIs) experiences in planning
same-day surgery show that operating room caseloads vary from day-to-day
and from one hospital to another. Rules of thumb for determining same-day
surgical caseloads are somewhat suspect in their overall validity for a wide
variety of facilities. Although a hospital may find that it has a feasible average
of potential cases (as defined by procedure), the numerical caseload is not in itself sufficient to validate more than a simple hospital-based service.

Including patient criteria fo admission to the service gives more complete
data to the planner. It also helps in preventing development of facilities which
might be underutilized. Such criteria might be developed through resolution of
the following questions:

- How old is each patient?
- How many of the selected patients have secondary diseases like hyper-
tension, diabetes, coronary damage, sickle cell anemia, etc?
- How large is the hospital service area and where do the selected patients
live?
- Is the patient's residence rural, suburban or urban?
- Where is the patient's residence in relation to the attending surgeon's of-
fice?
- Does the patient have a responsible adult at home to provide postopera-
tive observation and care?

Patients are not automatically candidates for same-day surgery simply because
of the type procedure to be performed or because they are relatively healthy.
Some low risk patients may live in rural areas without rapid accessibility to a
surgeon's office or to a hospital, precluding care of surgically induced complications. Some patients may not have responsible adults at home who can

provide intelligent postoperative care and observation. This is particularly important when the patient is very young or elderly. Patients may live in densely populated urban areas where trensportation to the hospital or to the physician's office is difficult. Many patients are pain-free at the time of discharge from the same-day surgical facility, but they can become uncomfortable by the time they approach their homes. If the method of transportation is subway, bus or train, some patients may be disqualified as candidates for same-day surgery.

Considering these factors, we conclude that not all hospitals can justify the development of a same-day surgical program which will yield high utilization rates. Some hospitals may find the satellite same-day facility as the best answer to meet their particular service area needs. These facilities have the capability of bringing care closer to where patients reside and work. A patient origin study may help the hospital identify the residences of its potential same-day surgical caseload and establish a need for the development of a remotely located but hospital-operated satellite. Such satellites do not necessarily provide a new service but merely extend the service arm of the hospital to a larger segment of the population. This concept is, of course, in direct opposition to the thinking of those who feel that same-day surgery belongs in a full-service hospital facility.

Determining the proper hospital-based program will vary with the scope of the hospital service area, the general age of the patient population, and the variable modes of living and socioeconomic composition of the hospital's patient population.

Once a reasonable and valid patient load is identified, the hospital should take the next step and survey its existing facilities, provided that data demonstrate the need for a campus-based service. The first consideration is the hospital's operating room suite and its staff. Initial questions to be raised include:
- How many times does an elective case get "bumped" from the schedule?
- Does the hospital's operating room suite accommodate a trauma service?
- Are anesthesiologists available to administer inhalation anesthesia to same-day patients, or will the surgeon be asked to use local anesthestics in order to maintain the operating room schedule?
- Will the anesthesiologist be available to screen preoperative patients on the day of surgery, and the morning prior to surgery?
- Will the anesthesiologist accept responsibility for discharging patients from the recovery room to their homes?

Negative answers to many of these questions may be sufficient reason for the hospital to abandon the idea of involving the operating room suite in its same-day planning.

Space

The modern operating room suite is designed for major surgical procedures. The large rooms, conductive flooring and extensive anesthesia equipment far exceed the requirement for same-day programs. Such factors cannot help but result in higher costs, which is in direct opposition to the same-day surgical concept.

Manpower

The scheduling of anesthesiologists will be done on a priority basis in the hospital operating room. Priority is given to major surgical cases which are urgent or emergent. In general, short-stay surgery receives less services from the anesthesia staff because of the lack of available manpower.

Scheduling

We all know that wait-list scheduling means accepting an operating room from a few weeks to as much as six weeks in advance. For surgeons contemplating short-stay surgery on patients requiring diagnostic procedures (to ascertain the presence of cancer), such as on some D&Cs, this concept is not well accepted. Yet, the gynecologist is the surgeon most often forced to accept wait-listing, since he frequently chooses the inhalation type of anesthesia. For this reason, gynecologists are the greatest utilizers of same-day surgical programs.

On the other hand, the oral, plastic, eye, ear, nose and throat surgeons will often choose to by-pass wait-listing for operating room time by using local anesthestics on their patients. Admittedly, many of their patients would normally receive local anesthetics, even if other services were available. However, our studies indicate that the percentage of cases completed by these same surgeons using local anesthetics would be considerably lower than one would imagine if an alternative choice of anesthesia were readily available. These surgeons are the high utilizers of same-day surgical programs. Surprisingly, many expressed a desire for inhalation anesthesia services versus local methods if an alternative choice were readily available. Hospitals are forewarned, then, to study the preference of their surgeons for local versus inhalation anesthesia, and the availability of these services in the operating room before deciding to use the suite for same-day surgery. In a formalized same-day program, the routine use of local anesthesia will increase the patient's postoperative recovery period, since preoperatively, many of these patients receive sedation.

The Movable Schedule

The surgeon who accepts wait-listing his patient for operating room time has absolutely no guarantee that his patient will not be "bumped" from the schedule by complicated, urgent or emergent procedures. The result can mean delaying the short-stay surgical patient. Sometimes a "bump" can be severe enough to move the case completely off schedule. In the latter instance, the patient is scheduled for another shift, or even another day.

The same-day patient, caught in the problems of the movable schedule, may end up needing sedation to keep him anxiety-free during this waiting period, thereby, increasing the effects of his anesthesia and prolonging his recovery time. It is not uncommon in such instances for the waiting surgeon who will perform a short-stay procedure to be asked to release the anesthesiologist, and to administer a local anesthetic to his patient. The request may be made because the anesthesiologist has been delayed or reassigned and the surgeon will lose his scheduled time to operate if he does not utilize another type of anesthesia. Planning should be directed toward identifying these potential problems before the operating room is designed for the same-day surgical service.

PROGRAMMING FOR FLOW AND FEAR

We believe that programming for a hospital service or department should be done on the basis of flow and fear. By this we mean that the program will not change the nature of the hospital's operating room or its staff. The operating room will remain a critical care area of the hospital, and the staff will remain committed to working efficiently in a stressful environment, making the recovery room less than ideal for the same-day patient who will remain, until he has awaken from the effects of anesthesia, and until he is "street ready" for discharge. Generally, the patient responds positively to the concept of same-day surgery. Nevertheless, it is best to plan the program negatively, from the position that the patient will remain happy with the new service *until* he sets foot inside the hospital. The normal fear of the unknown and apprehension about what could happen are certain to be experienced by the patient. The program must move smoothly to keep the patient's fear to a minimum.

Speed Is Essential

The faster the patient moves through the program, the less time he has to worry about his impending situation. The longer the time before surgery, the greater the need for sedation to prepare the patient. Downtime then from admission to actual surgery is critical. Flow should be smooth, rapid and as uneventful as possible.

The flow pattern to be accomplished is:
1. THE ADMITTING PROCESS with
   - Socioeconomic data collection
   - Consents/signatures
   - Arm-banding/securing of valuables
   - Development of the medical record
   - Care of companions
2. PRESURGICAL SCREENING
   - Laboratory work
   - Chest film
   - Electrocardiogram
3. PATIENT UNDRESSING
   - Locker, toilet facilities
   - Securing of dentures/prosthesis
   - Dressing in hospital attire
   - Transfer to wheelchair or stretcher
4. HOLDING
   - Preoperative care
   - Anesthesia clearance
   - Drug or intravenous administration

The problem of effecting a smooth admission process for the same-day surgical patient in the hospital setting can break down at several points.

The first problem may arise when the patient is required to have a chest x-ray. It may put him in contact with patients who are in poor health, augmenting his own fears of "what could happen." If the department has an outpatient waiting area, the problem is diminished. Any delay in taking the patient's chest film can increase his anxiety.

Conversely, the movement of the patient to the radiology department can be a benefit to the hospital-based service. Patients need to undress for chest films, and radiology departments usually have adequate dressing areas. The patient can be given a patient gown and cover robe to wear, secure his clothing in a bag, and be transferred with ease to the operating room.

Getting the patient undressed and caring for his belongings are difficult tasks for the hospital-based service to perform. The easiest, but most costly, method is to admit the patient to a nursing unit bed. Justifying the cost of personnel services, linen, and housekeeping becomes difficult for some hospitals. An alternative, often chosen, is to undress the patient in the operating room. This additional service, carried out by operating room staff in a supposedly controlled environment, leaves much to be desired. Use of the staff's locker room facilities is especially undesirable for esthetic reasons and because it violates the staff's need for privacy during rest periods.

Unequivocally, we recommend that the patient be brought to the operating room in the same manner as any other patient. Dressing should remain outside of the suite. As a concession, practice has shown that the operating room staff does not mind having the patient redress in the recovery room when he is deemed "street ready." Nevertheless, the controlled environment is destroyed, and the procedure cannot be advocated because it violates the principles of surgical technique.

Holding

Keeping the patient in a nonthreatening environment prior to surgery is the only way to eliminate the need for preoperative sedation. Most hospitals do *not* have a holding area in their operating room suites. Stretcher spaces in the recovery room, may, in some hospitals, be allocated for this purpose. A last resort, but unfortunately the most commonly chosen, is the operating room corridor.

The location of the holding area in relation to the operating room suite can be problematic for the anesthesiologist who needs to evaluate the patient preoperatively. If he must leave the suite in order to see the patient, he will encounter a problem in maintaining proper surgical attire. Program planning should address itself to the resolution of these problems.

PROGRAM PLANNING FOR THE RESOLUTION OF THESE PROBLEMS

Freestanding and satellite facilities are planned to resolve these problems, accommodate rapid flow of patients, and to provide spaces with assigned nursing personnel who provide the following services:
1. Complete the preoperative check-in process (including vital signs).
2. Carry out preoperative orders.
3. Start an intravenous feeding to maintain an open life-line.
4. Apply a blood pressure cuff to follow the patient through to recovery room.
5. Complete preoperative skin-site preparation.
6. Attach monitor leads to the patient.
7. Secure clothing and valuables.
8. Assist the anesthesiologist in preoperative examination.
9. Remain with the patient until transferred to surgery.

Planning for the provision of these same services in a hospital-based service (utilizing existing facilities) is tricky at best and will result in some kind of compromise. Such problems are most easily resolved with a same-day surgical department.

If the results of study of potential patients, services and staff are positive, one should be ready to make the final recommendations regarding the type of formalized program that should be developed by the hospital. The three choices are: simple service, independent department or satellite.

Determining the Number of Needed Operating Rooms

An operating room has 6 to 6 1/2 hours of actual operating time (for inpatients) in each eight-hour shift. Using the day shift for a baseline and assuming that the same-day surgical patient should be off the table by 2:00 P.M. (in order to recover and leave the facility no later than 5:00 P.M.), fewer cases can be scheduled than if the census were all inpatients. The hospital can plan to move five same-day surgical type patients through the room. Two rooms should be reserved for a ten case daily schedule. In summary, in same-day surgery planning, one room equals five cases. The exception will occur if patients are to be scheduled for surgery after 2:00 P.M.

We further advocate a simple same-day hospital-based service to meet patient needs if only one room is needed. Additional facilities, such as the allocation of beds outside the operating room suite, may not be considered as financially feasible. If ten patients per day are to be served, the need for some facilities external to the operating room suite will be necessary and can be considered feasible. Hospitals with potential caseloads of more than ten patients per day should be contemplating the development of a hospital-based or remotely located satellite facility, that is, if they anticipate overall future growth in the patient census.

Developing the Hospital-Based Same-Day Surgical Department

Certain elements, other than operating rooms, are needed for the same-day hospital-based surgical department. They include:
1. Holding/recovery spaces with possible induction area.
2. Dressing and toilet areas for patients and staff; staff spaces to provide for direct egress into sterile area.
3. Supply spaces for:
   a. clean goods
   b. sterile goods
   c. soft goods.
4. Janitors' closets.
5. A room (in the operating room suite) equal in size to one OR for the storage of portable equipment.
6. Clean-up and reprocessing facilities.

Portable equipment is expensive and does not tolerate handling very well. Replacement parts are difficult to obtain and, even in an improved economy, are not readily available. Improper handling and constant movement results in miscalibration of some equipment and breakage in others. If the hospital is planning to develop a same-day surgical department that is not directly adjacent to the operating room suite, sharing fragile portable equipment will create other problems than those mentioned. Portable equipment used for surgery should remain, according to proper principles of surgical asepsis, within the confines of the surgically clean environment where it will be used.

The most neglected area of space planning in the design of operating room suites is the lack of space for storage and safekeeping of portable patient care equipment. Planners of same-day surgery should remain alert to this problem to avoid repeating this costly error in space allocation.

Instrument and equipment processing facilities for a same-day surgical program may be shared with other hospital departments. Yet, instruments used by specialists who most frequently work in this setting are fragile, precious, not easily replaced, expensive and usually in need of some hand-processing. Therefore, some provision for the care of this equipment and reprocessing should be made in the department, unless experience has proven that central processing is nonproblematic. A high speed autoclave, of the type to process a single dropped instrument, is required. The need for larger autoclaves can be met from other hospital departments. A variety of scopes will be used in the same-day surgical department. Processing is usually by the bacteriocidal solution immersion method. If scopes are to be cleaned within the department, space for the immersion carts should be provided as well as a clean-up sink with oversink faucets for cleaning the lumens.

Mechanical-Electrical Considerations

Converting hospital trauma or outpatient clinic treatment rooms for the use of nonflammable anesthetics usually requires renovation. National Fire Protection Association (NFPA) Codes for Anesthetizing Locations apply to hospital and independent same-day surgical facilities. Some are unaware that isolation circuitry, monitors and transformers are necessary in the construction of same-day surgical rooms as well as for major surgery. Little attention has been paid to the Codes including those for gas alarms, grounding outlets, air-conditioning systems, humidity controls and gas shut-off valves. It is true that conductive floors may be eliminated when rooms are constructed for the sole use of nonflammable anesthetics. But many people assume that all other safety features can also be disregarded for the same reason. The safety features explicitly outlined in the NFPA Codes are not affected by the type of anesthesia to be used. Same-day surgery requires the use of many types of electrically operated equipment. Malfunction can cause patient or personnel burns, heart arrhythmias or fires. Hospital liability for resultant complications is of concern.

Air exchanges and humidity controls are required by the Codes not only to minimize static electricity but also to control the growth of pathogenic organisms. Asepsis is not obsolete for same-day surgery. Emergency power for operating rooms is necessary as well. The installation of grounding outlets and their proper use in operating rooms prevent patients and personnel from burns or other injuries resulting from malfunctioning equipment. Policy should dictate how such safety precautions should be carried out, and under what situations ground wires should be attached to furniture and equipment. If anesthetic gases (either flammable or nonflammable) are to be used, machines should be equipped with scavenger devices to protect personnel from resultant harm, including sterility and abortion.

The widely held concept that the surgical environment and safety features for same-day surgical operating rooms are different from those of general hospital operating rooms, is incorrect. The principles and the HEW-accepted NFPA Codes are the same for both types of suites. Why have planners decided that the structure of the operating room can change? Because the patient returns home after surgery rather than to a hospital bed.

Advocates of the development of freestanding same-day surgical facilities have argued that the cost of operating room construction is considerably less than those designed for a hospital. Such statements are certainly suspect. The cost of conductive flooring is insignificant compared to the total cost of all other required safety features. It is true that same-day surgery can be performed comfortably in rooms smaller than those needed for major surgery, resulting in lower square footage costs for construction. But a four room freestanding facility neutralizes the saving in the construction of ancillary facilities to become a million dollar fully-equipped structure.

The patient's postsurgical residence has no relationship to the requirements of his operative environment. As planners, we are deeply concerned that misunderstanding of what constitutes the proper surgical environment will cause a proliferation of same-day surgical facilities—both within and outside the hospital—which have none or few of the safety features recommended and tested by the NFPA after years of study and evaluation. Until they are proven otherwise, these regulations should apply not only to hospitals but also to freestanding facilities. Most hospital emergency rooms are not constructed to meet these codes and conversion to same-day surgical use should be preceded by renovation for code conformation.

Unquestionably, health planners seeking legislation for the regulation of same-day surgery should be concerned with a double-edged approach: one that affects hospitals as well as developers. Public health and safety is the concern at hand. Perhaps the best mechanism to accomplish review and approval for the planning process rests with the already functioning State Health Departments which license health care facilities and approve plans for construction prior to groundbreaking. Beefed-up regulations and supportive legislation are needed to give the State Health Departments the "teeth" they need to enforce proper standards for the construction of same-day surgery.

Part II
Hospital Programs of Ambulatory Surgery

In Part II actual case studies of successful hospital programs of ambulatory surgery are presented. Each chapter is a paper that was presented at recently held national conferences directed by the American Academy of Medical Administrators.

Alfred S. Frobese, M.D., chief of staff and director of surgery of Abington Memorial Hospital, describes the development of the "short-stay procedures" unit of that hospital in Abington, Pennsylvania. He regards ambulatory surgery and short-stay surgery as synonymous terms.

Dr. Frobese has been the program co-chairman of the three most recent AAMA conferences on ambulatory surgery, and has provided much leadership in our ambulatory surgery efforts. Each audience that has heard Dr. Frobese has been highly impressed with the description of the overall ambulatory surgery program at Abington Memorial Hospital. Dr. Frobese presents the background, problems and resolutions that evolved in this unit. He gives a full summary of all the major areas of ambulatory surgery at Abington Memorial Hospital.

The second hospital case study presented in Part II depicts Santa Barbara Cottage Hospital in Santa Barbara, California. Mr. Rodney J. Lamb., hospital administrator, describes the formal ambulatory surgical program of Santa Barbara Cottage Hospital. Emphasizing the dignity of the patient in preparing him for surgery, Mr. Lamb delineates how a completely self-contained unit was constructed immediately adjacent to the health care facility of Santa Barbara Cottage Hospital. In this way, each area of ambulatory surgery has been tailor-made for patient care. The entrance and all the bookkeeping procedures are separate from the inpatient section of the hospital. A complete separation of ambulatory surgery patients and inpatients is maintained.

Douglas D. Hawthorne, assistant administrator of Presbyterian Hospital of Dallas, Texas, developed a case study which is presented in Chapter 8. Drawing upon his past several years of experience, Mr. Hawthorne details the cost issues, types of procedures, and the full range of key issues in ambulatory surgery.

Chapter 9 provides a description of the case study of Phoenix Baptist Hospital in Arizona. The major organizational issues, background and tables illustrating the overall dynamics are presented by J. Barry Johnson, administrator. Assistant administrator for fiscal affairs, Robert Raatjes, describes the major cost issues that relate to the practice of ambulatory surgery at the Hospital. He shows the impact on average length of stay as a result of taking on a program of ambulatory surgery.

In Chapter 10 the Canadian experience in ambulatory surgery is discussed by J. D. Manes, M.D. Outlining the individual features of ambulatory surgery at Holy Cross Hospital, Dr. Manes tells how Canada's national health care system actually works.

L. Donald Bridenbaugh, M.D., associate director, Department of Anesthesiology, presents a case study of Virginia Mason Hospital in Seattle, Washington.

Part II offers a complete description of the major types of ambulatory surgery within hospital-controlled environments throughout the U.S.

Chapter 6
A Surgeon's View of Ambulatory Surgery

Alfred S: Frobese, MD

Health care providers are increasingly mindful of the escalating costs of health care delivery and of the increasing pressure for change. Most surgeons are not ignorant of these pressures. One innovation designed to increase delivery of surgical care at lowered or stable costs is ambulant short-stay surgery. In fact, the American College of Surgeons has sponsored workshops or study groups that have concluded that, in general, the concept is a good one. In the literature on ambulatory surgery, it has been stated that 20-40% of all operations now being done in most general hospitals could be eone on an outpatient basis at considerably lower cost. It has been demonstrated that this concept in no way lowers standards of patient care.

Surgeons, like physicians in general, are reluctant to change longstanding patterns which have produced good results. New ideas, therefore, are viewed with caution, which often is misconstrued as skepticism. However, in areas where hospital facilities are heavily utilized, the surgeon encounters difficulty in getting his nonemergent cases admitted. The uncomplicated hernia patient, for example, is competing with another patient with a more serious illness, resulting in weeks of waiting. In fact, in our hospital he might wait as long as eight weeks and then on the appointed day find he has been pre-empted by someone with a fractured hip. Thus the plans of both the surgeon and the patient are disrupted, and everyone is disgruntled. If it can be shown that the surgeon can apply the concept of short-stay to such cases with no sacrifice in the quality of care, I think he will become a most enthusiastic advocate of the concept.

I want to emphasize that the surgeon is not alone in this endeavor, as there are procedures of a nonsurgical nature performed by internists and radiologists which are suitably adapted to the short-stay ambulant concept.

My position is to confirm the rationale of the concept that ambulatory short-stay surgery, without diminution of quality of care, is valid and, further, that added dividends may result—other than better utilization at lower cost for those patients who are treated in such hospital-based units.

The program at Abington Memorial Hospital started in 1970. A brief review of this experience may serve to dispel many of the misgivings physicians, administrators, and patients might have.

The concept of a short-stay or "in-and-out unit" was not original. A large university hospital in Philadelphia had started such a unit months before, and we were aware of Dr. Reed and his co-workers who had established a freestanding unit with the same objective. In the past, the modus operandi at Abington Hospital for surgical patients not requiring major operative procedures, but needing general anesthesia, had included 40-48 consecutive hours of inpatient, and often mainly custodial, care. For example, patients were usually admitted at noon on the day prior to the scheduled procedure in order to allow the house officers an opportunity to obtain a history, perform physical examination, and order the indicated laboratory tests. The following day, the operation was performed, and the day after the operation, the patient was discharged from the hospital. This pattern was solidly established—as I suspect it is in many hospitals—because of the belief that close observation the night after the operation would either prevent complications or allow them to be spotted rapidly.

The "Blue Plans" considered that if a patient could be discharged at 5:00 P.M., that hospital day was an unnecessary and, therefore, a nonreimbursable day. Patients having procedures in the operating suite under local or regional anesthesia were handled in a more haphazard manner in that they were admitted by various routes, often via the emergency room which was involved in the pressing affairs of its own milieu. They were sent to the operating suite, disrobed and "prepped" where there were no facilities for either procedure, operated on, and returned to the emergency area for discharge without proper observation and instruction.

Most, if not all, of these patients could be handled through a short-stay unit which could coordinate their course. We started with a four-bed unit. Under previous practice there, four beds, utilized on a six-day per week basis, 24 hours per day, could have accommodated 12 patients per week. Under the new scheme, the same four beds staffed from 7:00 A.M. to 4:00 P.M. on a five-day per week basis with two patients per bed per day could accommodate 40 patients per week. We did not have four beds in the acute care section which could be spared; therefore a nonoccupied, nonincome producing area, a *solarium,* was physically altered with partitions, furnished with clothes lockers, chairs, recovery room type litters and a minimal nursing station with a capital outlay of $9,000. It was staffed by one nurse/clerk. Existing operating rooms and the recovery room were utilized.

Medical records were similar to the short forms used by the dental, and ear, nose and throat inpatient services of the hospital, and color coded for the short procedures unit to speed their collection. The completion of the history, physical and laboratory examinations 24 hours prior to admission to the unit was mandatory, since there was no time to obtain any of this after admission.

Cases suitable for admission to the unit were arbitrarily defined as those requiring no more than one hour of general anesthesia because of the postanesthetic recovery time required. If they were to be performed under local or regional anesthesia, they had to be the kind not ordinarily carried out in an office setting because of the magnitude of the procedure, or the special equipment, and skilled help required in the operating suite.

Cases under general anesthesia were scheduled first in the day. Such patients reported to the unit at 7:00 A.M. for operation at 8:00 A.M. This permitted adequate recovery time so that a second case, usually under local anesthesia, could be scheduled for that bed later in the day.

For the first 24 months our experience was successful enough that we enlarged the unit to seven beds with provisions for immediate expansion to 11 beds should it become necessary to meet the demand. The seven-bed unit has been operational for three months. It became apparent that the limited staff could not prepare seven patients for 8:00 A.M. operations. This has been corrected by scheduling three of the seven one hour later. With ten operating rooms the scheduling of seven short procedure cases at the prime time of 8:00 or 9:00 A.M. is not without friction. Needless to say, some surgeons object to starting long and difficult cases at 10:00 A.M., particularly if they never need the short procedure unit. However, it has not proved to be an insurmountable problem. Usually there is some leeway, and eventually the surgeon who objects to starting his list later in the morning because of short procedure cases has an occasion to use the unit for his cases and then becomes sold on the idea.

We have now reached a level of 200 patients per month processed through the unit. Eighty-five percent of these are surgical, and 15% are medical or diagnostic. We expect that the volume will reach 250 patients per month in 1976. Gynecologic procedures were not scheduled through the unit due to its limited capacity, until it was enlarged this year. In the first 60 days of booking gynecologic procedures, 58 were scheduled. In the enlarged unit, the staffing had to be increased. This now consists of a receptionist/clerk, one registered nurse and one licensed practical nurse.

The following are the procedures that we presently find suitable.

1. General surgical procedures include:
   a. Hernias, both pediatric and adult. Pediatric hernias have long been carried out on a 24-hour stay without difficulty. Uncomplicated adult hernias have presented no problem in the unit. Repair of recurrent or

bilateral adult hernias should not be performed because of technical difficulty, the need for prolonged anesthesia, or the increased incidence of postoperative problems.

b. The breast lump suspected to be benign but requiring excision for confirmation. Why should the patient with a probable fibroadenoma or cystic mastitis be admitted for an extensive workup, such as before a radical mastectomy, when, in fact, such workups should be reserved for the patient who has obvious or "likely" breast carcinoma. If the lesion thought to be benign proves to be a carcinoma, there is no evidence that mastectomy 24-48 hours subsequent to biopsy is deleterious to the patient.

c. Varicose saphenous veins requiring only high ligation or several low ligations are suitable. We do not recommend ligation and stripping operations in the unit because of their time consuming nature.

d. Large subcutaneous lesions such as lipomas, fibromas or lymph node excisions which are too extensive for office management.

2. Plastic surgical procedures include skin lesions which require plastic revision, some skin grafts, or those lesions which are too extensive for office management.

3. Orthopedic procedures are mainly fracture rereductions under general anesthesia, digital amputations, bunions, ganglia, tendon transplants or repairs, or those procedures requiring use of tourniquets.

4. Proctologic procedures include fissures, fistulas and any surgery not above the anorectal line; the latter because of frequency of acute urinary retention following surgery.

5. Neurosurgical procedures ideally include "carpal tunnel syndrome"—often bilateral.

6. Urologic procedures include cystoscopies in children, circumcision, vas deferens ligations, meatotomies.

7. Otolaryngologic operations include myringotomies and selected adult tonsillectomies.

8. Gynecologic procedures done are perineotomy, hymenectomy or hymenotomy, D&C, diagnostic and therapeutic culdoscopy, laparoscopy, and laparoscopy with tubal ligation.

9. Medical procedures include selective aortography and arteriography in normotensives, and invasive needle biopsy techniques not considered suitable for office practice.

As our experience increases, the list expands.

Approximately two patients per month have valid reason for transfer into the acute care section of the hospital. I have had two breast excision cases found to have carcinoma which required transfer; one laparoscopy was complicated by bowel perforation; one therapeutic D&C was complicated by uterine perforation; and one hernia developed a hematoma in the recovery room necessitating re-exploration. Most of the transfers are indicated because of unanticipated intraoperative problems, which require prolonged anesthesia. Therefore, these patients have not recovered sufficiently for discharge by 4:00 P.M.

About two-thirds of the patients processed through the unit have general anesthesia. To date there has been no anesthetic complication requiring resuscitative measures.

There have been very few problems after discharge. One surgeon who did 125 adult hernias through the unit had to make a house call on one patient to catheterize him for acute urinary retention. Several breast biopsies and two large lipoma excisions developed hematomas of the wound. All had been drained at surgery and developed the hematoma after the drain had been removed. A 24-hour hospital stay after surgery would not have prevented these problems. In short, we have been unable to find fault with this management.

The idea that overnight observation for this type of patient is a *must* simply does not hold up in our hospital, considering the limited number of night nursing personnel and the time they spend tending the needs of the more seriously ill on their floor.

Surgeons have been enthusiastic about their ability to schedule patients for the operating room on a lead time of 2-4 days.

Anesthesiologists at our hospital were, at first, concerned that in their first preoperative visit with the patient about an hour before operation, a proper preanesthetic evaluation would be difficult because of a lack of needed information. This, however, has not been a problem; surgeons or referring physicians have been relatively accurate in their selection of cases for the unit. So far no one has tried to "sneak" a patient with marked cardiac disability or electrolyte imbalance through the system.

Patient acceptance of the concept has been high. When assured that they will not likely suffer harmful consequences at home, patients enjoy the comfort and security of their home. Perhaps an added dividend is the presence of one's spouse extending sympathy. Regardless of the hospital's achievement in culinary skills, food still tastes better at home where it is usually served when one is hungry instead of at 5:00 P.M.

Administration has been pleased as the major third-party payers in our area have reimbursed the hospital at levels comparable to its other divisions. The unit does not operate at a profit, but it does not function as a "loss leader" either. Since the hospital's goal is to serve the community's needs within its resources, such a unit serves this end.

Third-party payers should be eager to participate in these programs as they are not confronted with charges for three days of purely custodial care.

Does this concept really reduce cost? We think so. Our patients are charged the same amount as inpatients for the use of the operating room, laboratory or x-ray work, anesthesia and surgeon's fees, but they pay only an hourly fee ($5) for the actual time spent in the unit. This averages out to $12 per patient. Patients having general anesthesia and, thus, requiring essentially a two-day stay under the old scheme would have had a $90 room charge. I also believe there is a hidden advantage in this program since the patient is worked-up by his own surgeon or internist who knows him and is, therefore, more likely to order the preoperative laboratory and x-ray examinations which he believes are indicated. Under the inpatient system, often the patient is admitted and a conscientious, diligent house officer who does not know the patient's past or present problems orders more tests than necessary and, perhaps, some that were done previously as an outpatient.

I am also convinced that this experience is influential in shortening inpatient postoperative stays. We note that patients having other major procedures, such as cholecystectomy, are being discharged earlier as it is established that they do well at home.

I wish we could get the internal medicine physicians to discharge some of their patients earlier. I am convinced that the ritual of a specified minimum of days for certain "diseases" should be abandoned, and that each case should be treated on an individual basis.

In summary, I heartily recommend this concept. Our experience indicates that it is a method of extending surgical care to more patients at a lower cost, without sacrificing quality. It helps the surgeon by allowing him to schedule procedures on shorter notice and reduce competition with emergency admissions and medical services for inpatient beds. The program emphasizes the value of preadmission testing and makes us take another look at our old "norms" for postoperative stays.

Chapter 7
Outpatient Surgery: The Importance of the Planning Phase

Rodney J. Lamb

It is extremely helpful to those of us in the health care industry to share our experiences, particularly when a relatively new concept such as outpatient surgery is involved. At Santa Barbara Cottage Hospital we sought the advice and experience of others in planning our outpatient surgery program. Now we are pleased to share the information about the planning and preopening activities which led to the establishment of this new service to our community. We hope our experience will prove helpful to others.

INITIAL IMPETUS

At the outset, one might ask what initiated our planning for an outpatient surgery program. Primarily it was the reports we read and heard about this concept, particularly about the group in Phoenix, Arizona. The idea appeared sound from every aspect: the psychological factors relating to the patient; the high standard of patient care; the convenience to surgeons; the speed of patient recovery; the avoidance of separation of patient and family; and the reduced costs of delivering this type of health care. We were also aware of the trend of outpatient services throughout the country. The American Hospital Association statistics indicate that in the decade from 1963 to 1973, community hospital outpatient visits per capita increased 94%.

Our particular needs also stimulated a serious search for possible solutions. The hospital had recently been almost entirely rebuilt, but the operating room schedule was rapidly expanding. Concern was frequently being voiced by surgeons and anesthesiologists that the surgical area needed expansion. Even under ideal circumstances expanding a surgery area is very costly. At Santa Barbara Cottage Hospital the operating room is on the second floor and is bounded by exterior structural walls. Expansion of the surgical space would be exceedingly expensive.

We were also experiencing congestion in our emergency room, which was relatively new. Case volume was increasing sharply, and we were scheduling outpatient surgery through our emergency room. The preparation and recovery phases of these patients were causing ever increasing congestion in our emergency department. The growing facility problems of our emergency and operating rooms gave us the impetus to look seriously for solutions. A specialized facility for outpatient surgery was becoming a clear and attractive alternative.

In summary, we became increasingly convinced by our own needs, the trends in the health care industry, the logic of the concept, and the demonstrated success elsewhere that outpatient surgery had a place in our hospital. To our way of thinking this was a favorable climate for embarking on a planning project.

The First Steps

The planning phase began a full year before the actual opening of the facility. We were, of course, well underway as a result of reports we heard about other units. We sought and readily found members of our medical staff enthusiastically willing to study this new concept with us. After general conversation, one of the first things we did was to visit the Phoenix Surgicenter®. On successive trips the facility was viewed first hand by the president and past president of the medical staff, both surgeons; several anesthesiologists; the president of the Board of Directors; and the administrator. We were given exceptional cooperation by Drs. John Ford and Wallace Reed and their staff. Viewing their facility first hand, watching it function and having many of our questions answered was the most important activity during the planning of our unit. As a result, there are significant similarities between our unit and the Phoenix Surgicenter®.

On return, we requested designation of a special committee representing the surgical specialities and anesthesiology. The entire concept was discussed in depth by this ad hoc committee. In due course a recommendation came forth to the executive committee of the medical staff endorsing the establishment of an outpatient facility within the existing hospital framework. The executive committee's recommendation to proceed was directed to the Board of Directors. At this level approval was readily forthcoming.

An architect was commissioned to begin the schematic drawings for the unit. These plans were reviewed by the surgical and anesthesia staff and operating room supervisor. When agreement between design and function had been reached, working drawings were begun.

The outpatient surgical unit is accommodated in an existing single story structure. It is a separate building located on the hospital grounds. Fairly extensive remodeling was needed to convert the building to its new function.

Significant planning also occurred during the construction phase. We held a meeting with all hospital departments to explain the concept of outpatient surgery. We showed the plans and described in detail how the unit would work. We found these meetings beneficial; they promoted understanding and enthusiasm for the concept.

Operational Plans

We also formed ad hoc operational planning groups of varying composition. The make-up of these groups depended on the particular matter being discussed. There were, however, some constants in these groups: an anesthesiologist, the unit's head nurse and representatives of administration.

Following are the kinds of policies and procedures covered by this operational planning group. These topics comprise a kind of shopping list and may be of considerable importance to those in the planning phase of outpatient surgery.

First and foremost, we discussed the organizational relationship of the unit. It is a separate facility, and, organizationally, it is a separate department. From the beginning our goal has been to create an outpatient surgery unit as part of the hospital that would be relatively autonomous. It is neither part of nursing, nor part of the main operating room; it is separate.

We logically proceeded to the next basic consideration, direction of the unit. We requested and readily received the cooperation of our anesthesiologists. One staff member serves as part-time medical director of the unit on a salaried basis. We also have a head nurse with the usual responsibility for direction of those employed in operating the unit. In fact, the unit is separate both physically and organizationally.

The next planning concept *was* the criteria for patient selection. We decided that the final decision would rest with the anesthesiologist. If there is a question, he, in consultation with the referring surgeon, decides on the appropriateness of scheduling. In practice, according to our anesthesiologists, nearly all of the patients on whom procedures are performed fall in the Anesthesia Society of America (ASA) classification Groups I and II.

In the planning phase we also discussed scheduling and the processing of patients, charges and payment policies. When the patient presents evidence of approved insurance coverage, a $35 advance payment is requested. When there is no recognized insurance coverage, full payment is requested in advance.

Only two routine laboratory procedures are required on all patients: a dip stick urinalysis and a hematocrit determination. Both are performed the day of surgery by a registered nurse as part of the preoperative processing of patients.

Additional laboratory work requested by the surgeon or anesthesiologist is performed in our laboratory or another prior to the day of surgery.

The medical record form involved significant discussion. A new form was designed. Related topics of use, numbering system, completion, transcription and filing were decided. On completion of the operative procedure the record is now handled by the central medical records department in the usual manner.

Staffing of the unit, of course, was extremely important. Logically, an incremental basis of staffing was established. As the volume of the unit increased, staffing was augmented according to a predetermined formula. In our unit, with two operating rooms, we have maximum capability—under ideal circumstances—of scheduling approximately fourteen cases per day. We cannot overemphasize the importance of staffing and the selection of personnel for this unit. We strive for qualities of exceptional motivation, enthusiastic interest, and a genuine desire to treat the whole patient from the beginning to the end of his stay. Personnel with these minimum qualities are indispensable to the success of our unit.

How were personnel selected? The head nurse interviewed and screened those interested in working in the unit. Final selection was on a group basis. The applicant was interviewed by all the nursing personnel and anesthesiologists. Where group identity and esprit de corps are so important, this mechanism has proved valuable.

The printed material included preadmitting forms, an operative record form, a patient information brochure, a patient instruction card, and a preopening news media release. Figure 7:1, a simplified floor plan showing the flow of patients, is the result of structural and operational planning.

Getting Underway

In keeping with the usual delays one expects with any construction or remodeling program, we opened between two and three months after our target date. Our first cases were scheduled November 13, 1973. Immediately before the opening we engaged in some of the customary activities which we thought important. An open house was planned for all employees, medical staff, and our auxiliary. Invitations were also extended to the employees of the doctors' offices. We thought it extremely important for those who would have contact with the unit through scheduling and related activities to know how it functioned.

As predicted, the start of the unit was slow. The case load did build gradually but predictably. The growth has continued to the present. We are now very close to capacity (based on our present Monday through Friday 40 hour weekly schedule). The statistics shown in Table 7:1 reflect the surgical caseload

FIGURE 7:1   FLOOR PLAN

Patient entrance is shown adjacent to waiting area. Flow of patients is generally counter-clockwise to the laboratory, dressing room, preparation, O.R., recovery, discharge waiting and finally departure via the designated exit. Area without designation is used for a function unrelated to outpatient surgergy.

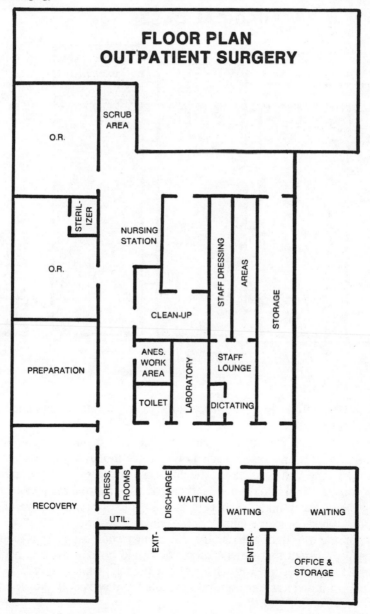

TABLE 7:1   HOSPITAL SURGICAL CASELOAD

While there has been a slight decline in cases performed in main operating room, the hospital's total surgical caseload has increased 21% between 1972-73 and 1974-75. Cases in outpatient surgery have increased 53% between first and second years unit has existed.

SURGICAL CASES

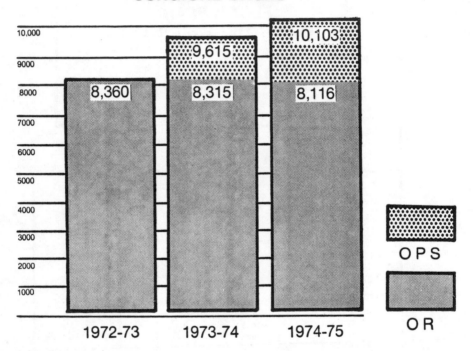

of the hospital and its two components, the main operating room and the outpatient surgery unit.

While there are real financial benefits, the cost of providing comparable surgical service in this new unit or in the conventional area is essentially the same. The time that is required, the supplies consumed, and the amount of professional staffing needed are nearly identical. The greatest opportunity for savings is in streamlining, such as in laboratory procedures. By far, the most significant saving is in the elimination of overnight stays.

Within one month of opening the unit a suggestion came from the general surgery department that general surgeons should boycott the unit because of expressed dissatisfaction with charges. Fortunately, sanity prevailed. An explanation of how rates were set was requested and provided. Apparently, the matter was adequately handled because the surgeon who was particularly concerned is now one of the heavier users of the unit. Perhaps this experience attests to the fact that regardless of intent or effort, you cannot plan for everything.

The outpatient surgery unit has had the expected impact on case composition of the main operating room. Tables 7:2 and 7:3 reflect the changes in time and numbers. Figure 7:2 shows use of the facility by the surgical specialties of the medical staff.

TABLE 7:2   AVERAGE LENGTH OF CASES IN MAIN OPERATING ROOM

Figures show a significant increase each year, amounting to 12.8% between 1972-73 and 1974-75. Effect of removing minor cases is apparent.

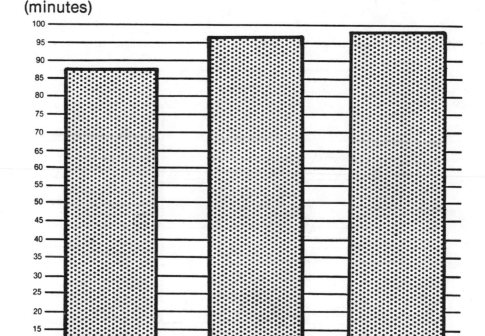

TIME
(minutes)

| 86 | 94 | 97 |
| 1972-73 | 1973-74 | 1974-75 |

Response

The response to our outpatient surgery unit has been outstanding. We feel our objectives have been met. Our experience to date attests to the psychological impact of this unit on the recovery of the patients. Their early return to usual activities has also been substantiated.

Expressions of satisfaction from members of our medical staff and from patients are frequent and enthusiastic. A scrapbook is being kept in the unit. The

TABLE 7:3   MAJOR CASES IN MAIN OPERATING ROOM

Again a reflection of concentration of activity in main operating room.

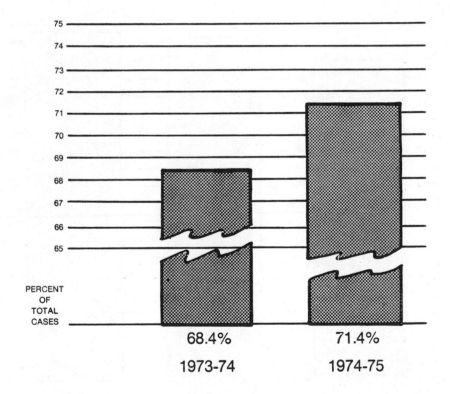

(EXPRESSED AS PERCENT OF TOTAL CASES)

warm response that has come from the patients is truly remarkable. And the gifts of candy and other food attest further to the satisfaction of those we serve.

A registered nurse contacts all our patients by phone the day following surgery. Inquiry is made as to how the patient is feeling and whether he has any questions. The nurse does her best to provide answers including advising the patient to contact the surgeon if there appears to be reason to do so. We feel this contact is an excellent procedure. Not only can sound professional advice

FIGURE 7:2   USE OF OUTPATIENT SURGERY BY SURGICAL SPECIALTIES

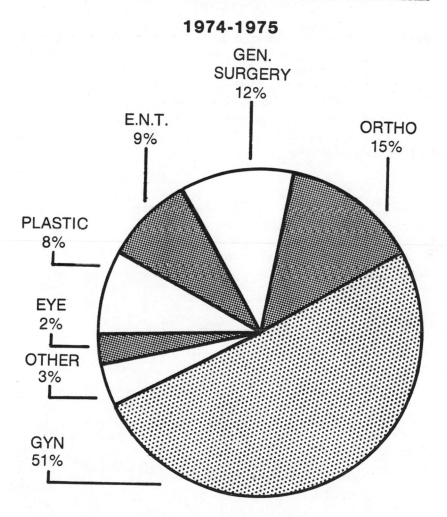

be given to the patient, but we have the ability to follow reaction to the unit on a daily basis. The public relations response to this procedure is outstanding.

What happens to patients who have procedures done on Friday? If we wait until Monday to call these patients, we lose contact because they have gone back to work or resumed their usual activities. Friday's schedule is recorded on cards. One of the nurses takes the cards home with her and contacts the patients from home on Saturday, since our unit is only open Monday through Friday. It is one more example of the attitude of our personnel that is reflected in patient care.

CONCLUSION

Our conclusion is that if the need for an outpatient surgery unit can be justified, we heartily commend it. We are delighted with our first years of operation. However, we do strongly recommend a substantial period of advance planning. We have endeavored to describe one such effort. The details may well differ in each case. The key is involvement of those personnel who will function within the unit. The effort expended in intelligent planning will be more than repaid by the satisfaction of a well-conceived unit offering patients high quality surgical service.

Chapter 8*
Hospital-Based Unit
Improves Utilization

Douglas D. Hawthorne

A day surgery program at Presbyterian Hospital of Dallas has raised the quality of care, reduced the duplication of services, and lowered costs. In the past four years, more than 7,500 patients have received care in the day surgery unit.

Presbyterian Hospital of Dallas, a 500-bed, general, acute, not-for-profit community hospital, opened in 1966. In 1971, the hospital census averaged over 90 percent on a seven-day-week basis, and patients had to wait two to three weeks for elective surgical procedures. To improve utilization of surgical beds, we opened a day surgery unit.

PLANNING

The first step was to design a model to evaluate costs in a day surgery unit. (See Figure 8:1.) Three basic steps were involved in this planning process: development of a list of one-day surgical procedures; approval of a payment process with third-party reimbursement; and design and construction of an area for the day surgery unit, including policies and procedures for the unit's operation.

The one-day stay cases first were developed through local hospital and Professional Activity Study (PAS) statistics as well as through medical staff input. A list of 35 surgical procedures was developed and approved by the medical staff's operating room committee. These approved procedures traditionally had been one-night and two-night stays in the hospital that could well be done on a one-day basis. The list later was expanded and the 10 most common as well as the other procedures that have been performed in our unit are listed in Table 8:1.

*Reprinted, with permission, from *Hospitals, Journal of the American Hospital Association,* Vol. 49, October 1, 1975, pp. 62-65.

Some of these procedures, such as hemorrhoidectomy and cast changes, have been performed only once or twice, while others, such as dilation and curettage, tonsillectomy and adenoidectomy, and dental extraction are performed almost daily. The hospital's operating room committee approves all day surgery procedures. All procedures listed in Table 8:1 previously were performed at Presbyterian Hospital on a conventional basis, and most procedures are listed in the PAS regional manual as having stays of at least one to two nights. Many of these procedures are still performed on a conventional basis because some physicians will not utilize the unit and some patients' emotional or physical conditions prohibit their use of the unit.

To ensure reimbursement, the administrator wrote to the hospital's 10 major insurance carriers, describing the proposed day surgery service and requesting third-party support of the program. The response was 100 percent favorable, an indication that reimbursement would be forthcoming on claims submitted for day surgery patients. A day surgery patient was categorized as an inpatient and counted as one patient day. Since we began, only one claim (a university student group plan, which disallowed any stay under a 24-hour period unless it was at the student health center on the university campus) has been denied. Although Medicare does not reimburse for one-day service on an inpatient basis, this policy may change to allow Medicare patients the option of day surgery.

CONSTRUCTION

Early in 1971, a seven-bed experimental day surgery unit was constructed in a 1,200-square-foot area in the lower level of the hospital. It was approximately 75 feet from the entrance to the main operating room and recovery area, convenient to transport patients and near back-up emergency services. Because of the high occupancy level in our conventional beds, we built a new unit rather than convert existing beds. Policies and procedures were developed to detail the patient flow process and to delineate the responsibility of all departments involved.

Because of the one-day stay concept, it was necessary to develop policies to provide a tight control over the patients for the eight-hour hospitalization period. Some examples of these policies are that all patients scheduled for day surgery must report to the unit at 6:30 a.m. on the day of their scheduled surgery to allow the anesthesiologist time to visit the patient prior to surgery, to give the patient time to settle in the new environment, and to adjust if a change in the surgery schedule is made; that a patient cannot be discharged from the day surgery unit without a written discharge order from the attending physician; and that patient charges are centralized and delivered to the business office before the patient is discharged so that the patient has a complete bill when he leaves.

ADMINISTRATION

The concept of day surgery is simple. The program is operated under the direction of the hospital administration and of the nursing service, with medical direction from the operating room committee. Patients are admitted in the morning, have the required surgical procedure, and return home that afternoon.

Patients scheduled for day surgery report to the hospital the day before their scheduled surgery to complete preadmission papers, to have laboratory work and x-rays performed, to visit the day surgery unit for familiarization, and to receive instructions from a registered nurse. On the day of the scheduled surgery, the patient reports to the unit to be prepared for surgery. Following the preoperative medication, the patient is transferred to the main operating suite. After surgery, he is sent to the main recovery room area and then returns to the day surgery unit until discharge.

FIGURE 8:1   MODEL TO EVALUATE PATIENT COSTS IN A DAY SURGERY UNIT

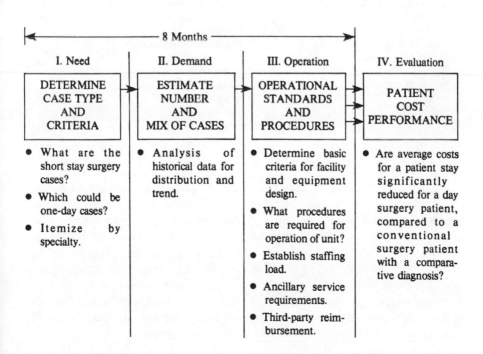

TABLE 8:1   DAY SURGERY PROCEDURES, 1971-75

Ten Most Common Procedures

Dilation and curettage
Cystogram and pyelogram
Tonsillectomy and adenoidectomy
Myringotomy
Laryngoscopy
Dental extraction
Breast biopsy
Bilateral oscular muscle procedure
Scar revision

Other Procedures

Voluntary interruption of pregnancy	Tubal ligation
Blepharoplasty	Circumcision
Toenail removal	Redundant tissue removal
Lipoma removal	Nevus removal
Plate (bone) removal	Neuroma removal
Metacarpal wire removal	Neck lesion excision
Polyp excision	Eye cyst excision
Hymenal ring lesion excision	Partial keratectomy
Nose reduction	Nasal septum repair
Bronchoscopy	Ligament repair
Herniorrhaphy	Ptosis
Tear duct probe	Otoplasty
Brachial arteriogram	Augmental mammoplasty
Curettage of maxilla	Ligament repair
Skin graft	Transurethral resection
Ulnar nerve transplant	Hymenotomy
Salpingogram	Nasopharyngoscopy
Carpal tunnel	Cast change
Exam under anesthesia	Hemorrhoidectomy

All day surgery cases are performed before noon so that patients have adequate time to recover before discharge. Several studies have indicated that the average time for a patient to go through the complete day surgery process is approximately seven hours, which includes an average time of 65 minutes in the operating room, 55 minutes in the recovery room, and the remainder of the time in the day surgery unit itself. Presbyterian's day surgery unit is open from 6:30 a.m. to 6:00 p.m., Monday through Saturday. Patients who are not fully recovered by 6 p.m. and who need further observation are transferred to a conventional nursing unit for an overnight stay. With the emergence of more diagnostic work, expansion to two shifts is being contemplated.

During the first three years of operation of the seven-bed unit, 5,014 patients were accommodated (80 percent occupancy), which included 13 medical services and 130 participating physicians. Approximately 96 percent of the patients were discharged the same day. Of all the patients admitted, 94 percent received a general anesthetic.

Because of the overwhelming success of the experimental seven-bed unit, a new 20-bed unit was opened in mid-1974. (See Figure 8:2.) With the 17 existing operating rooms, we anticipate that the unit will have at least an 80 percent occupancy rate. Each room in the new unit has air, oxygen, vacuum, television, a nurse call system, and a toilet facility for each two patients. The unit also has a consultation room for the completion of preadmission work, a small specimen collection area, a small pantry area for convenience-type meals, a large nurses' station, and a family waiting room. The rooms can easily be used for a conventional patient requiring overnight hospitalization. A two-month study in the new unit indicated that approximately one-third of all cases performed in 14 categories were done as day surgery. (See Table 8:2.) Certainly, there is potential for increased utilization on a day surgery basis.

TABLE 8:2 SURGICAL PROCEDURES PERFORMED AT PRESBYTERIAN HOSPITAL, APRIL-MAY 1975

		Conventional		Day surgery unit	
Procedure	*Total*	Number	Percentage	Number	Percentage
Dilation and curettage	177	117	66%	60	34%
Tonsillectomy and adenoidectomy	162	99	61	63	39
Cystoscopy and pyelogram	149	115	77	34	23
Myringotomy	88	36	41	52	59
Voluntary interruption of pregnancy	69	13	19	56	81
Tubal ligation	52	31	60	21	40
Dental extraction	31	29	94	2	6
Breast biopsy	29	24	83	5	17
Laryngoscopy	11	5	45	6	55
Scar revision	10	5	50	5	50
Blepharoplasty	8	5	63	3	37
Cast changes	7	5	57	3	43
Circumcision	5	3	60	2	40
Ocular muscle resection	4	2	50	2	50
Total	802	488	61%	314	39%

FIGURE 8:2 TWENTY-BED DAY SURGERY UNIT

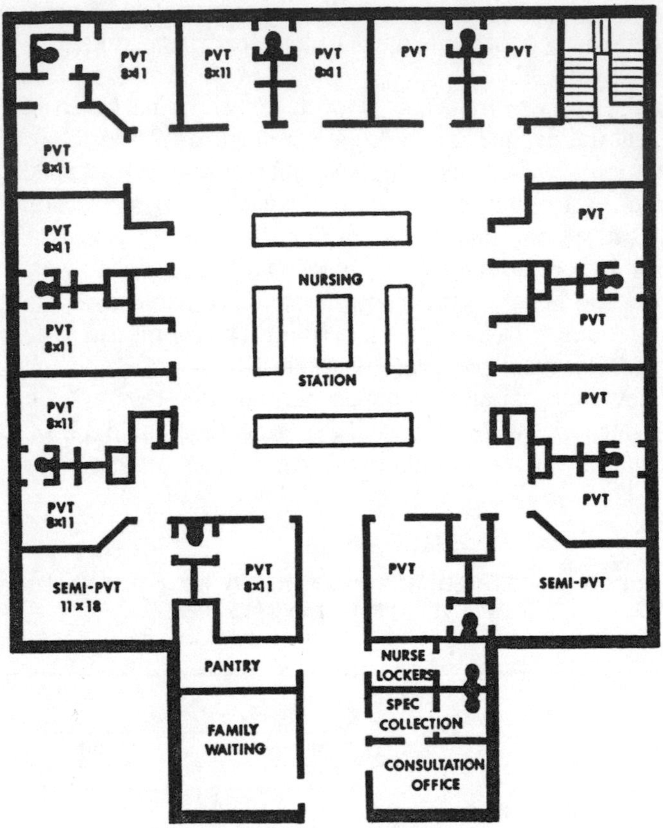

In addition to a more efficient utilization of the hospital's surgical beds and a high level of patient satisfaction, the day surgery program lowered costs by approximately $100 per case compared to conventional surgery. Over four years, more than $550,000 has been saved. The largest savings is in the reduction of the daily service charge, which includes room and board. Costs in other areas, such as x-ray, laboratory, pharmacy, and central service, also have been reduced. Comparison of conventional surgery costs and day surgery costs raises the question of possible overutilization of services in conventional cases. Certainly a closer examination should be made of daily services. The longer a patient remains in the hospital, the more services he will receive and the more it will cost. In over 600 cases studied, day surgery cases created substantial savings.

When the day surgery unit first opened, a study indicated that physicians were ordering more medications, supplies, laboratory tests, and x-ray procedures on patients who were going to be in the hospital at least two nights than on patients who were going to be in the hospital for only a day. When this apparent overutilization of services by conventional patients was brought to the attention of the medical staff, the discrepancy between the two types of patients narrowed. The most significant reduction in cost is the room charge, because the overnight stay is eliminated. For example, a surgical procedure performed on a conventional basis averages two nights in the hospital, a $130 charge; the same procedure done on a day surgery basis costs $47 for the one-day stay.

The total number of surgical procedures done annually at Presbyterian Hospital has increased steadily in recent years. However, before the day surgery unit opened in 1971, there were long waiting periods for elective surgery: plastic, oral, ear, nose, and throat surgical patients had to wait two to three weeks and gynecologic patients had to wait for up to five weeks. The increase in the hospital's surgical cases was a result of the increase in operating rooms from 9 to 17 in 1974. This increase reduced the waiting time and redistributed all types of cases, which brought back some surgeons who had been taking their cases to hospitals with shorter waiting periods. At the same time, more physicians are realizing that procedures that traditionally kept patients in the hospital for two to three days now can be done in one day with greater convenience and satisfaction to the patient.

Chapter 9
Ambulatory Surgery: A New Look at an Old Concept

J. Barry Johnson

A freestanding ambulatory surgical facility located in close proximity to a hospital and owned and operated by the hospital is feasible and desirable for the average hospital in America today.

Early postoperative discharge of patients from hospitals began in 1941 and was popularized by Dr. D. J. Leithauser. Before early ambulation, patients frequently died from pulmonary emboli, pneumonia and other complications. Surgical recovery was slow, not from the surgical trauma, but from the prolonged period of inactivity and bed rest. If without surgery, a healthy person were put to bed for a week and given narcotics at intervals, it would take him several weeks to recover from this experience.[1]

If early postoperative discharge is not new (some hospitals have been doing it for 20-25 years), then why all the fuss and concern over it now? There are several reasons why hospitals and physicians are now looking at freestanding ambulatory surgery facilities very closely.

1. Hospitals are being pressured by patients, government and other third parties to provide needed services at lower costs.

2. Hospitals are encouraged by various programs such as utilization review, medical audit, and PSROs, to reduce the patient's length of stay.

3. The current depressed economy and high unemployment forces the patient to think more about having surgery and being away from his work.

4. There is a desire to maximize convenience for the physician who can in one stop make inpatient rounds, obtain test results on patients, fulfill inpatient surgical commitments, and perform his scheduled outpatient surgery.

5. Certificate-of-Need laws are forcing hospitals to look for other alternatives such as outpatient facilities instead of adding beds.

6. Patients want to maximize convenience by fewer rules and regulations due to the minor nature of surgery (e.g., in an outpatient facility, the patient's family is allowed to accompany him to the preoperative and recovery areas—a courtesy that is unthinkable for inpatient surgery cases).
7. Because of a more predictable surgery schedule of an outpatient facility, physician and patient are not subject to cancellation for emergencies or delays by prolonged, complicated major surgical procedure.
8. The patient's psychological outlook on medical care is changing. Today patients are better educated about health problems through the media. Twenty years ago, the patient entering the hospital for surgery was frightened by the unknown. He was told he might be hospitalized for several weeks, which he interpreted to mean he would be sick. When he came out of surgery, his fears were focused on minor discomfort, which he quickly magnified into real pain. The narcotics he received only prolonged the recovery period. In contrast, the patient of today who knows he will be up and around the afternoon of surgery is relaxed and less fearful, requiring little postoperative medication.

In 1975, the Orkand Corporation, a research group doing work for the Social Security Administration, began a study of independent and hospital owned ambulatory facilities. The purpose of the study is to provide information to the Social Security Administration on whether independently owned ambulatory facilities will receive Medicare approval.

Table 9:1 shows that: Pennsylvania has thirty ambulatory surgery centers all owned by hospitals; Ohio has fourteen, California has thirteen, Florida, Illinois, and Texas have ten each; forty-one states have a total of 204 centers; thirty-eight states have 149 hospitals with centers; twenty-three states have centers that are independently owned; seventeen hospitals are now planning and building centers; and six nonhospital owned centers are now being planned and built.

TABLE 9:1 AMBULATORY SURGICAL CENTERS BY STATE

State	Hospital Owned	Non-hospital Owned	Total
Alabama	2	—	2
Alaska	—	1	1
Arizona	2	6	8
Arkansas	1	—	1
California	7	6	13
Colorado	1	—	1
Connecticut	2	1	3
Delaware	1	2	3
Dist. of Columbia	1	—	1
Florida	8	2	10

Georgia	3	—	3
Hawaii	—	3	3
Idaho	—	—	0
Illinois	6	4	10
Indiana	3	4	7
Iowa	4	—	4
Kansas	2	1	3
Kentucky	4	1	5
Louisiana	1 ·	—	1
Maine	—	—	0
Maryland	1	—	1
Massachusetts	3	2	5
Michigan	5	1	6
Minnesota	4	1	5
Mississippi	—	—	0
Missouri	1	3	4
Montana	3	—	3
Nebraska	1	—	1
Nevada	4	1	5
New Hampshire	—	—	0
New Jersey	1	—	1
New Mexico	—	—	0
New York	3	2	5
North Carolina	5	1	6
North Dakota	—	—	0
Ohio	13	1	14
Oklahoma	2	—	2
Oregon	1	1	2
Pennsylvania	30	—	30
Puerto Rico	—	—	0
Rhode Island	—	1	1
South Carolina	—	—	0
South Dakota	—	—	0
Tennessee	5	—	6
Texas	4	6	10
Utah	3	—	3
Vermont	1	—	1
Virginia	3	—	3
Washington	3	4	7
West Virginia	—	—	0
Wisconsin	5	—	5
Wyoming	—	—	0
Total	149	55	204

Total Ambulatory Surgery Centers in Operation. 204
Total Ambulatory Surgery Centers Planned by Hospitals. 17
Total Ambulatory Surgery Centers Planned by NonHospitals. 6

Note: Information provided by the Orkand Corporation, Silver Spring, Md.

In 1971, when Phoenix Baptist Hospital began to plan its own freestanding ambulatory surgery facility, it had 119 beds and was performing approximately 3,000 operations on an inpatient basis. At that time, only one other freestanding unit existed in Phoenix, which was over 6 miles from our hospital. In 1971 Phoenix had 581,000 persons, so we thought a second unit at Phoenix Baptist Hospital was a good idea. Today, Phoenix has 800,000 people, and there are five ambulatory surgery units in the city. In April 1973, our freestanding ambulatory surgery unit opened with four operating rooms. Since that date, there ve been 3,600 operations performed by more than 90 physicians.

The Baptist Hospital and Medical Center campus is located in the northwest section of Phoenix with good access by freeway and four-laned roadways. The ambulatory surgery facility is located approximately 100 feet from the main hospital building and has its own entrance and exit patient flow patterns, parking facilities, support facilities, and physicians' offices. It is connected to the hospital by a covered walkway.

The ambulatory surgery unit is located on the first floor adjacent to the outpatient x-ray, laboratory and pharmacy, which provides support to this unit. The surgery unit is made up of three basic areas (Figure 9:1).

1. The admitting, business office, area includes:
   - A reception-waiting area
   - A business office, cashier area
   - Patient dressing and shower area (male and female).
2. The preop, surgery and central supply area includes:
   - Six-bed preop holding area
   - Four operating rooms
   - O.R. scheduling and control area
   - C.S.R. and storage area
3. The recovery-discharge area includes:
   - Thirteen-bed recovery area
   - Discharge, patient pick-up area

Structurally, the ambulatory surgery unit is very similar to the inpatient surgery unit. However, it does not need all the expensive emergency-type backup equipment normally found in inpatient units. It also enjoys the economics of shared central services with the hospital such as: nursing services, payroll and accounting, housekeeping, purchasing, engineering, laboratory, x-ray and pharmacy (backup), administration, billing, linen and laundry, personnel, and medical records. These savings are reflected in patient charges.

Medical direction and responsibility for the unit comes from a standing committee of the medical staff, which reports directly to the executive committee of the medical staff. The committee meets every other month to review the utilization and quality of medical care in the unit.

FIGURE 9:1 OUTPATIENT SURGERY BUILDING FLOOR PLAN

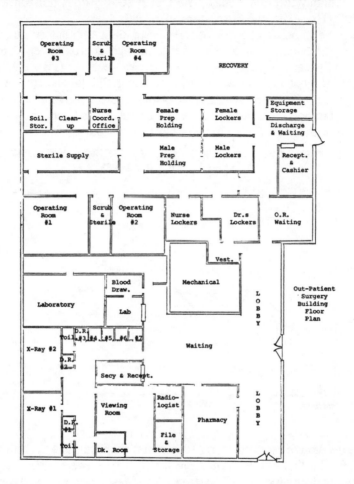

The method of providing anesthesiology coverage for the unit is very important. Presently, the private group of anesthesiologists working in the hospital provides coverage to the outpatient unit. Determining how many anesthesiologists a unit needs depends upon how anesthesia is practiced in a community, the outpatient surgery volume, and how many hours the anesthesiologists want to work. Generally, one anesthesiologist can handle up to 175 outpatient procedures per month. For a volume of 175 cases per month with a setup similar to ours, staffing should consist of one supervisor, five operating room and recovery room nurses, one orderly, one aide-CSR technician, and the equivalent of 1.5 business office clerk/receptionist. The total is 9.5 full-time employees. The unit is normally open from 7:00 a.m. to 5:00

p.m., Monday through Friday. The unit presently does not run a Saturday schedule. However, the hospital inpatient unit does.

Since the Phoenix Baptist Hospital freestanding ambulatory surgery facility opened thirty months ago, we have performed approximately 3,600 cases. Presently, we are averaging between 9-11 cases per day (Figure 9:2). A normal utilization of an ambulatory surgery room in Phoenix is approximately 5-6 cases per day. There are several reasons for our present overall utilization rate. The most important is that there are five ambulatory surgery units in Phoenix, and one of these units is only three blocks from our unit.

FIGURE 9:2   GROWTH OF SURGICAL PROCEDURES IN OUTPATIENT AMBULATORY FACILITY

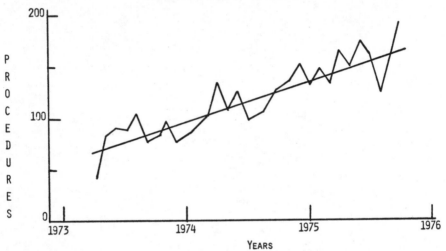

The division of cases by type of surgery has changed since the unit opened in 1973. Of the first 650 cases done in the unit, 50% were ob/gyn cases, 22% were general surgery, and 17% were EENT cases. Orthopedic and plastic surgical procedures totaled 6%; urologic and oral cases totaled 5%.

The last 650 cases were distributed as follows: gyn, 33% EENT, 31%; orthopedic and plastic, 19%; and general, 16%.

The distribution of all cases since opening the unit is shown in Table 9:2. The drop in gynecologic cases can be explained by the opening of an ambulatory surgery unit within the same office building, which is occupied by the group of five ob/gyn physicians who were active at our hospital. The rise in EENT, orthopedics and plastic cases can be explained mainly by the education of these physicians as to the safeness of the unit for patients.

Table 9:3 shows the sixteen most common procedures (in 1975) in the order of their frequency. There were 175 different types of procedures performed in the outpatient facility. Figure 9:3 shows the growth pattern in six-month intervals since the facility opened in April 1973. Table 9:4 indicates the patient distribution by age category. More than 75% of the patients are between 14 and 65 years of age. Tables 9:5 and 9:6 indicate that approximately 90% of all ambulatory surgery patients receive general anesthesia, and about the same percentage are discharged the same day.

Tables 9:7 and Figures 9:4 and 9:5 show the effects of the ambulatory surgical unit on inpatient procedures, average length of stay, and admissions, respectively. As one might expect, the number of inpatient minor operations is drastically reduced. There is no effect on the volume of inpatient major procedures. In addition, by moving the short-stay cases from the hospital to the ambulatory surgical unit, the average length of stay for all hospital admissions increases.

TABLE 9:2 COMPARISON BY SURGERY CLASSIFICATION OF TOTAL PROCEDURES SINCE OPENING APRIL, 1973

Gynecology	1,373	40%
Ear, Nose, Throat	811	24%
General	595	17.5%
Orthopedic	224	6.6%
Eye	182	5.4%
Plastic	129	4%
Other	87	

TABLE 9:3 GENERAL STATISTICS FOR AMBULATORY SURGERY UNIT

Total procedures (April 1973—October 1975)	3,602
Average number of procedures per month (1975)	151
Total number of physicians using facility (1975)	83
Number of different procedures performed in facility	175

16 MOST COMMON PROCEDURES IN ORDER OF FREQUENCY

1.	D&C	295
2.	Tonsillectomy or T.&A.	236
3.	D&C suction	141
4.	Laparoscopy with or without tubal coagulation	134
5.	Breast biopsy	101
6.	Excision masses (various locations, all specialties)	85
7.	Adenoidectomy	84
8.	Excision lesions (various locations, all specialties)	80
9.	Muscle recessions or resections	73
10.	Ganglionectomy (GS, ortho)	42
11.	Laryngoscopy	37
12.	Septoplasty	23

13.	Removal hardware	23
14.	Excision or partial excision of toenails	17
15.	Vasectomy	16
16.	Scar revision	16
		1,403
Other		405
	TOTAL	1,808

TABLE 9:4   PATIENT DISTRIBUTION BY AGE CATEGORY

Age	Number of Patients	Percentage
0-13 years	702	20.6
14-65 years	2,585	75.8
65 years & over	121	3.6

TABLE 9:5   COMPARISON OF GENERAL AND LOCAL ANESTHESIA IN AMBULATORY SURGERY FACILITY

Type of Anesthesia	Times Used	Percentage
General	3,044	89.5
Local	365	10.5

FIGURE 9:3   SIX MONTH COMPARISON OF NUMBER OF PROCEDURES SINCE FACILITY OPENED APRIL 1973

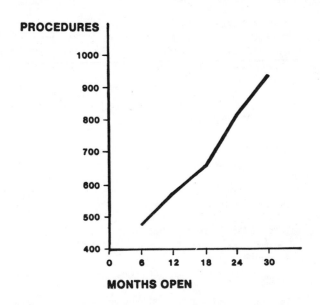

TABLE 9:6   COMPARISON OF NUMBER OF PATIENTS NEEDING HOSPITAL ADMISSION vs. PATIENTS GOING DIRECTLY HOME AFTER AMBULATORY SURGERY

	Number of Patients	Percentage
Scheduled Hospital Admission	415	12
Unscheduled Hospital Admission	29	1.5
Discharged Home	2,953	86.5

TABLE 9:7   COMPARISON OF AVERAGE LENGTH OF STAY FOR HOSPITAL INPATIENTS

Years	Average Length of Stay (in days)
68/69	5.9
69/70	5.7
70/71	5.5
71/72	5.6
72/73*	5.5
73/74	5.8
74/75	6.0

* Outpatient Surgery Opens

FIGURE 9:4   OUTPATIENT SURGERY FACILITY IMPACT ON PATIENT PROCEDURES

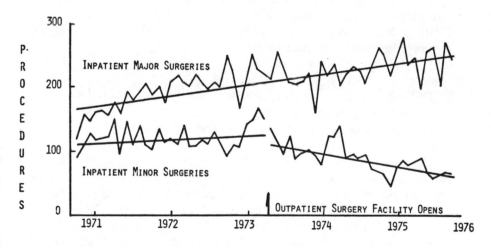

FIGURE 9:5   RATE OF INCREASE IN ADMISSIONS TO HOSPITAL FOR LAST 7 YEARS

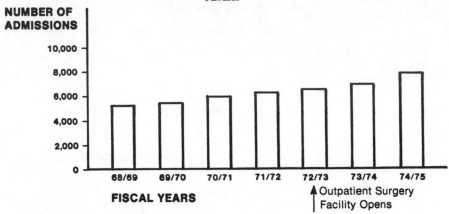

In summary, freestanding ambulatory surgery facilities are feasible for most hospitals today if several of the following factors are present or provided for:

1. The unit should be built distinct and separate, but close to the hospital and doctors' offices.
2. There should be ready availability of x-ray and laboratory facilities.
3. The savings of lower operating costs must be passed on to the patient.
4. The hospital should have average utilization of inpatient OR facilities with average distribution of minor cases in specialties as previously discussed (gyn., EENT, ortho., and plastic).
5. Strong State Certificate-of-Need laws with regulations designed to hold down the number of inpatient hospital beds.
6. The physicians must believe in early postoperative discharge for their patients.
7. The patient must be shown the value of early postoperative discharge *before* his surgery and of cost savings by using the outpatient facility.
8. There should be restrictions of types of procedures done in the unit to include *only* minor elective cases.
9. There should be availability of inhouse anesthesiologists for the unit.

In this period of rapidly rising costs, a freestanding ambulatory unit has a lot to offer the patient, the physician, the third-party payers and the hospital.

There is generally no valid reason to keep a surgical patient in a hospital environment any longer than needed for recovery from anesthesia. Although it is always difficult to fight the traditions of the past, the rewards of change are more than worth the effort to those involved.

Notes
1. Paul T. Lahti, "Early Postoperative Discharge of Patients," *Michigan Medicine,* September 1970, p. 755.

Chapter 10
Financial Aspects of Ambulatory Surgery

Robert Raatjes

In 1970 when Phoenix Baptist Hospital was seeking approval from the local Health Planning Council to build an ambulatory surgery facility, its main justification for the proposal was the anticipated cost savings to patients. Twenty surgical procedures, which were considered the most common, were selected to be performed in the outpatient facility. These procedures included tonsillectomy, adenoidectomy, D&C, mass and lesion excisions, etc. It was determined that 980 operations of the 20 selected procedures had been performed within the hospital during a 12-month period. Each of the 980 patients had been in the hospital for either one or two days, and the total charges billed to these 980 patients were computed. Then, based upon the proposed all-inclusive charge concept, the charges which would have been incurred by these patients for outpatient surgery were calculated. The patient savings on these 980 procedures would have been $135,196. Based upon the projected total number of procedures which would be performed in the ambulatory surgery facility during its first year of operation, it was estimated that the saving to the community would be in excess of a quarter of a million dollars during the first year. (See Table 10:1.)

Obviously, some of the projected savings to the community would result in lost income on the inpatient side of the hospital's operations. Since these procedures would be done on an outpatient basis, many would be transfers from those previously performed in the hospital operating suites. Since the hospital had been generating more revenue from these patients when they were hospitalized than when they became outpatients, there would be an immediate net loss in total revenue. But it was anticipated that the growth in outpatient surgery and the increase in major surgery in the operating room would very quickly more than offset the initial net loss in revenue. This proved to be true. The result is that most minor procedures are now performed in the ambulatory surgical facility, and almost all major procedures are performed in the OR.

TABLE 10:1   OUTPATIENT SURGERY SAVINGS TO PATIENTS

Actual inpatient charges incurred by 980 surgery patients who could have used outpatient facility	$ 246,556.
Charges which would have been incurred by these 980 patients in the outpatient facility	$ 111,360.
PATIENT SAVINGS ON 980 SURGERIES	$ 135,196.
Average savings per procedure	$ 138.
Projected number of procedures during first year of operation	2,000
Projected first year savings to community (2,000 x $138)	$ 276,000.

Note: Phoenix Baptist Hospital

Another interesting issue is that the average length of stay for the hospital's total patients showed an immediate *increase* when the ambulatory surgery facility opened. There were two reasons for this: (1) the minor procedures were replaced by major procedures in the hospital OR, which required longer stays; (2) the mere fact that the minor procedures were transferred to the outpatient center and were no longer considered as hospital admissions automatically inflated the total average length of stay for the hospital without any actual increase in the amount of time spent by remaining patients (Table 10:2).

TABLE 10:2   INCREASED LENGTH OF STAY BY REMOVING SHORT-TERM PROCEDURES FROM HOSPITAL ADMISSIONS

No. of Patients	Length of Stay	Patient Days of Care
500	1	500
1,000	2	2,000
500	3	1,500
500	4	2,000
1,000	5	5,000
1,000	6	6,000
1,000	7	7,000
1,000	8	8,000
1,000	9	9,000
7,500		41,000

Average stay of above mix	5.5 Days

Results of removing 500 one-day stays and 500 two-day stays:

Patient days of care	39,500
Divided by number of patients	6,500
= New average length of stay	6.1 Days

Note: Phoenix Baptist Hospital

The all-inclusive pricing concept was adopted for the ambulatory surgery facility. The current price list for this facility lists about 175 procedures which can be performed on an outpatient basis. There is a single all-inclusive charge for each procedure. There are no separate charges for drugs, supplies, room time, lab tests, etc. The patient, of course, still receives separate billings from the surgeon and anesthesiologist. The billing system is quite efficient from a financial administration viewpoint. Overhead is substantially reduced because all individual charge slips are eliminated; the patient knows what the hospital cost will be in advance; and billing the patient is greatly simplified. Since the patient knows the total hospital charge in advance, he is expected to pay upon arrival any amount over and above what insurance will pay. In every possible instance, we try to either verify insurance coverage or receive payment from the patient before the surgery is performed. There are, of course, exceptions; but a very meaningful result of this all-inclusive pricing concept is that the bad debt loss experience in the ambulatory surgery facility has been less than 2%.

Since its inception, the ambulatory surgery facility has been recognized by all insurance companies and Medicare for payment purposes. This has not been the case with freestanding outpatient surgical facilities that are not affiliated with a hospital. Private insurance carriers have been slow in recognizing such facilities for payment. Medicare is now conducting a study to determine whether or not they will pay for Medicare patients treated in an outpatient surgery facility which is not part of an overall hospital operation.

We had determined that the break-even point for our facility was approximately 150 operations per month; and it was anticipated that this break-even point would be reached at about the end of the first year of operation. In actuality, it took about two years to reach this point. For the past year, the number of operations performed each month has been well in excess of the 150 mark. One of the main reasons why the break-even point was not reached as quickly as anticipated was that the local health planning agency approved the construction of another ambulatory surgery facility in a medical office building within one mile from our hospital. It opened about six months after our facility opened. Whether or not such facilities should be permitted to be operated by groups not affiliated with a hospital, as far as quality of care is concerned, is an entirely separate question. But from a financial viewpoint, our experience has led us to conclude that a proliferation of ambulatory surgery facilities should not take place. The volume of surgery projected for our facility did not occur as soon as anticipated because another ambulatory surgery facility opened for business within the same vicinity, resulting in duplication of facilities.

If the concept of ambulatory surgery is truly going to save the community money, these facilities must have a sufficient volume to permit them to operate efficiently. Obviously, a proliferation of ambulatory surgery facilities will prohibit the efficiencies which can be realized.

Table 10:3 shows a summary of the operative revenues and expenses of our facility for the 12-month period ending June 30, 1975. During this 12-month period, 1,606 outpatient operations were performed, which was a little less than the amount needed to break-even. Consequently, a small net loss was experienced. The current financial results of the ambulatory surgery facility show a positive surplus.

In summary, from a financial viewpoint, Phoenix Baptist Hospital has benefited in many ways from the addition of the ambulatory surgery facility. The facility has now passed the break-even point and is generating a surplus for the hospital. The original minor operations which were transferred from the inpatient surgery department to the outpatient facility have been replaced by more extensive major operations, resulting in increased revenue for the hospital. Substantial savings have been realized by patients utilizing the ambulatory surgery facility, and Phoenix Baptist Hospital is providing a much needed service for the community.

TABLE 10:3   OUTPATIENT SURGERY REVENUE AND EXPENSES FOR TWELVE-MONTH PERIOD ENDING JUNE 30, 1975

Direct expenses:	186.630
Number of operations performed	1,606
All-inclusive patient charges	$ 186,630
Deductions from revenue	(3,265)
NET PATIENT REVENUE	$ 183,365
Salaries and wages (8 employees)	$ 63,475
Supplies	20,320
Other expenses	255
TOTAL DIRECT EXPENSES	$ 84,050
OPERATING SURPLUS AFTER DIRECT EXPENSES	$ 99,315
Indirect expenses:	
Employee benefits	$ 11,425
Depreciation, interest & insurance	68,365
Housekeeping and maintenance	16,285
General and Administrative	19,350
TOTAL INDIRECT EXPENSES	$ 115,425
NET OPERATING LOSS AFTER APPLICATION OF INDIRECT EXPENSES	$ (16,110)

Note: Phoenix Baptist Hospital

Chapter 11
Ambulatory Surgery in Canada

J. D. Manes, MD

Holy Cross Hospital was founded in 1882 by the Grey Nuns as a 4-bed hospital. Today it is a 533 acute bed general hospital, offering all community services and open heart surgery. It does not perform organ transplants.

Some seven years ago, the Sisters sold the hospital to the government and it is now a nonsectarian, community-owned hospital. Calgary, a city with a population of approximately a half-million, is located about 150 miles north of Great Falls, Montana. Calgary is known for a world famous stampede, which is the largest rodeo in the world.

The province of Alberta has four major industries: oil, beef, grain and health care. Alberta isn't unique in listing health care as one of its major industries. It is a fact for all of Canada. The history dates back to the early 1960s when the Canadian government decided that a socialized system of medical care was needed because the free enterprise system was not providing adequate medical care to Canadians.

A Royal Commission was formed. Chief Justice Hall, an eminent jurist with socialistic leanings, headed the Commission. For a year and a half, he toured the country and received briefs from every segment of the Canadian population. Finally, after two years, Justice Hall brought medicare to the Canadian people. Although ill-conceived, the system has been supported by wooly-eyed economists and the federal government.

When the Royal Commission was formed, the Canadian Medical Association told the federal government that Canada could not possibly afford this type of luxury. At the same time, the Canadian Institute of Chartered Accountants told the government the same thing. They cautioned that in 10 years it would be necessary to increase income taxes by approximately 20%, and it would be necessary to increase business taxes by approximately 50% to cover the cost of health care, as it was proposed by the Hall Commission.

The government didn't believe either group and proceeded. Since then, they have discovered that the accountants were almost on the mark, within about a million dollars. Approximately 20% of Canadian taxes goes to health care and its maintenance.

The Royal Commission recommended that there be free hospitalization and free medical care for all Canadians. They insisted that such care be universally available to all people, that it be comprehensive, include all services and be transferable from one province to another. Only the last condition was not met.

Health care is normally a provincial responsibility, so each province has a slightly different health scheme. Alberta, being a very conservative area, resisted the inroads of state medicine for many years. And it was only when our provincial politicians discovered that it was costing the taxpayers of Alberta some $94 million annually to stay out of medicare that they succumbed. The arrangements in Alberta are similar to those in Ontario; the other provinces vary slightly.

All medical fees are completely paid by the government — in this case, the Alberta Health Care Insurance Commission. The physician submits his diagnosis and charges (with a fee code)on an IBM card. This goes into the computer, and approximately six weeks later the physician receives payment for the service. This has resulted in the development of a total fee schedule for the medical profession. For example, the fee for an appendectomy in Alberta is $175, plus $29 for the anesthesia. It may appear to you that this compensation is too low. In fact, the physician has to do a lot of work. However, every visit and every service which is rendered to every patient is paid. As a matter of fact, there are provisions to opt out of medicare, but the government makes it very difficult to do so.

In Alberta all hospitals are controlled by the Alberta Hospital Services Commission. They don't pay all hospital costs, but they give a global budget within which each hospital must live. The patient's sole financial responsibility is to pay a $5 admission fee upon admission to a hospital. This is the last cash outlay. Frequently, patients don't pay the $5 fee, but legislation requires that three invoices or bills be sent them. It is obvious that trying to collect $5 three times is a definite loss.

The all-inclusive hospital admission fee of $5 covers the patient's room, every procedure, IVs, medications and operating room. There are no separate charges. A short time ago a young lad was admitted to the hospital, at which time his family diligently paid the $5 admission fee. Three days later the patient left the hospital with a $5,000 nuclear pacemaker in his chest. The $5 fee was obviously quite a bargain.

But to the hospital, this poses a real problem. The result of this socialized approach to medicine has been a longer length of stay in hospitals. From the patient's point of view it is understandable; he has paid $5 for a bed, comfort, room service, so he feels no rush to get out. From the doctor's standpoint, the sooner he discharges the patient, the faster he can admit another patient. It is not uncommon for a doctor to tell a patient he will be discharged on a Thursday, for instance, and for the patient to ask to remain until Friday for his own convenience. Once you take away any financial responsibility from the patient, you face this situation.

Along with longer lengths of stay has come increased utilization, particularly in laboratory and radiology services. The physicians must take responsibility for this, though patients often demand tests when they are admitted, and the physician is quite content to order all the tests that may seem even remotely pertinent. Many patients decide they might as well have an ECG, chest x-ray and upper GI series. The physician does not hesitate to order any radiological tests which might bear on the case only slightly. These practices increase the cost of treating the individual patient. Over the last 10 years, the government has naturally been concerned with this increase in health costs, and has considered ways of limiting it.

In Ontario the government decided to close a certain number of beds. According to my colleagues, they actually didn't close them; they transferred them into long-stay or chronic care, but they did reduce the active treatment beds to about 4-4.5 per thousand persons.

In Alberta the government has decided that it will control the situation by not building any more hospital beds. Presently there are 6.5 beds per thousand in Alberta, but they are maldistributed. Governments have thought it wise to build 30-bed hospitals in small towns, which are less than 50% full, and are filled mostly with flu and colds and, sometimes, pneumonia or occasional heart attacks. Most of the surgery comes into the main centers. The result is overbedding in smaller areas and underbedding in metropolitan areas of 4.5 per thousand.

The other method of control is by a global budget. The government will tell us exactly how many millions of dollars we have to operate with, including all operating expenses. Regardless of how many nuclear pacemakers we need to install, we will still have to live within the global budget. We do have a separate capital equipment budget, which amounts to about $365 a bed per year. At Holy Cross Hospital it amounts to approximately $175,000 annually, which we have available to spend on capital equipment. When some special need for equipment arises, the physician can submit a request to the Hospital Services Commission, which will fund it separately, if they feel it is worthy. Recently, we submitted a request for another cardiac catheterization laboratory because we had outgrown our old one. A short time later we were notified that they were indeed giving us $750,000 for a new cardiac catheterization laboratory.

The hospital has to react in some way to these global budgets and to the spiraling costs of health care. One of the methods, of course, is to cut back or to freeze present services. The other method has been to develop short-stay surgery. In Canada we don't have the problem that is prevalent in the U.S. of convincing Blue Cross of the importance of ambulatory surgery. Blue Cross only provides for preferred accommodations (private rooms, ambulance service, and drugs prescribed by physicians in excess of $25).

AMBULATORY SURGERY

We have learned from the American experience that it is indeed cheaper to use one-day surgery or short-stay surgery than to admit a patient for two or three days for the same procedure. In Canada, because of the system of global budgets, there is absolutely no way we can break down the overall figures in ambulatory surgery. We do not have to keep track of how many drugs each patient gets, or how much radiology. It's not important, and it would only increase our costs if we had to individualize the cost of all these services. Much experience in the U.S. has shown that it is bound to cost less to perform surgery on an ambulatory basis than on an inpatient basis.

We have had no trouble selling short-stay surgery in our hospital to doctors, because it means they can get their patients in faster, and they can do more procedures with that fee schedule as I described previously. They are quite happy with it. It has been more a job selling the concept to the patients, who have to be convinced to get up at 6:00 or 7:00A.M. and go to the hospital with nothing to eat, be operated on, and go home again, instead of being admitted for a couple of comfortable days. Our selling job has to be done on the patients, not the physicians.

Three years ago Holy Cross Hospital began withhfour ambulatory surgery beds, gradually increasing to eight, and then twelve. We didn't have enough space to have all the beds in one place until this fall when they were all contained in one area. I looked at our occupancy rate and saw the same phenomenon that existed worldwide: our obstetrical unit was only at about 55% occupancy. I took twelve beds from the obstetrical unit and turned them into a short-stay unit.

In 1972, with four beds, we did 872 surgical procedures. In 1973, going from four to eight beds, we did 1,257; and in 1974, with eight beds , and going to 12, we did 2,254 procedures. This accounts for approximately 22% of all our surgical procedures, and is quite a large percentage, compared with most hospitals.

The short-stay surgical unit runs about 94.8% occupancy. The only time there is not 100% occupancy is when an occasional patient arrives with a cold, or having eaten breakfast, despite previous instructions.

We have developed a list of 85 acceptable procedures to be done in the short-stay surgical area. This past year we added breast biopsy. We don't do

T&As because of different opinions among our medical staff. Among our ten leading procedures in the short-stay unit are D&Cs. In 1974 we did 168 therapeutic abortions. The second most common procedure is myringotomy, then, cystoscopics, incision of ganglion, incision of skin, and subcutaneous lesions, dental procedures, removal of orthopedic devices (such as screws), and cardiac catheterization. We expect cardiac catheterizations will increase considerably when we open our new cath lab later this year.

The short-stay area that we have is an open area, with stub walls. We use stretcher beds which are taken straight from the short-stay area of the operating room to our main operating room for procedures. The patients report in at 7:00 A.M. and are discharged by 4:00 P.M. If there are any who have to be retained after 4:00 P.M., we transfer them to another nursing unit. We manage this unit with two registered nurses and one clerk. We don't have to have the financial arrangements common in the U.S. We perform surgery until 1:00 P.M., except for dental procedures, which we only do until 12 noon. We have found in the past that the dental procedures seem to take considerably longer (as long as two hours). The recovery from anesthesia is therefore too long to do them any later.

Our anesthetists discourage the use of ketamine for short-stay surgical cases because of the problems that may result after the patient goes home. I had one incident where I used ketamine on a pair of twins; one went home and was fine, and the other began hallucinating. The mother became quite concerned. We have since discouraged the use of ketamine.

Our complication rate has only run at about 5 per thousand; and the greatest proportion of these complications has been breast biopsy which was found to be malignant. At Holy Cross Hospital we sort of rearrange the morning schedule in such cases. We proceed to do a radical, modified radical, or whatever the surgeon deems appropriate. The patient is then put into one of the nursing units. We don't close them up and readmit them at a later time.

In general, I think our system of short-stay surgery doesn't vary much from many others.

Chapter 12
A Hospital-Based Ambulatory Surgery Unit

L. Donald Bridenbaugh, MD

Virginia Mason Hospital is an approximately 300-bed general surgical hospital located in the center of metropolitan Seattle. All types of surgery including open heart, major neurosurgical procedures, and organ transplants are performed. It is located immediately adjacent and connected to a large multispecialty clinic of approximately 100 physicians. The particular motivation for the establishment of an ambulatory-surgery unit in our hospital was the shortage of hospital beds, and a community health planning agency which would not permit addition of more hospital beds because of the underutilized beds in nearby hospitals. Surgeons were waiting two to three weeks to schedule elective patients. The surgical suite was operating at 52% utilization. A newly constructed emergency room and recovery room were being utilized even less. The establishment of ambulatory surgery services was the obvious answer to the problem. In reviewing the type of facility which would best meet our needs, we considered the following:

1. *A freestanding unit* (such as the Surgicenter® in Phoenix), a specially planned facility solely for ambulatory surgery, offering the ultimate in potential efficiency and economy for both patient and surgeon. However, the price paid for this convenience was the cost of construction of duplicate facilities and duplication of personnel. With underutilized staff, operating rooms, and recovery rooms at Virginia Mason, this did not seem appropriate.

2. *A hospital-based satellite unit,* which offered the efficiency of a freestanding unit but with hospital back-up, standards and organization. Again, this called for duplication of facilities and personnel.

3. *An integrated hospital-based unit* which utilized existing facilities. This seemed to be the best answer to our problem.

105

The central elements for the functioning of an ambulatory surgery unit include: an admitting area and receptionist; a laboratory; an interview, scheduling, and examination area; a waiting room for both patients and individuals accompanying them; a dressing area; an operating area; and a postanesthesia recovery unit. All of these areas were apparently available in the hospital. Therefore, the short-stay surgical services of the Virginia Mason Hospital were inaugurated in March 1969. The unit was started and, like so many hospital-contrived units, was dispersed. The receptionist and interview area was in an unused emergency room space on the first floor south of the hospital; the admitting area was located on the first floor center of the hospital (in the hospital's regular admission area); the waiting and additional interview areas were located in the hospital's main entrance waiting room on the first floor center; the laboratory was on the second floor west of the hospital; and the operating room and recovery room were on the second floor east wing of the hospital. An additional receptionist and advanced scheduling area was located on the seventh floor of the adjacent clinic building. Needless to say, patients were inconvenienced, frequently lost, and the result was often a delay in the surgical schedule. Because these patients were receiving the same care as inpatients, the requirements for laboratory work-ups, hospital admission, and operating room charges were the same. We soon discovered that this was unnecessary and unjustifiably expensive.

For these reasons, patients were frequently dissatisfied, and surgeons began seeking other facilities for performing ambulatory surgery. The hospital then encouraged the development of a "package charge" for the most commonly performed surgical procedures—e.g. D&Cs, cyctoscopies, etc.—based on pertinent laboratory work-up as determined by the surgeon and the anesthesiologist; a man-minute charge for surgery based upon the personnel, equipment, and time required of operating room facilities. In order to eliminate the confusion and delay in the surgery schedule, written instruction sheets, informational brochures, and a specially designed receptionist area were developed.

In spite of these disadvantages, the unit functioned and flourished between 1969 and 1974 to the satisfaction of surgeons, third-party carriers, hospital administration, and most patients. Although patients realized they were being inconvenienced, they were likewise saving money.

A review of the service during the past five years shows the following:

1. *Surgical Procedures*—Although more than 300 surgical procedures have been proposed as appropriate for ambulatory surgery, gynecology, ENT, plastic surgery, and GU (Genital-Urinary) are the most common services utilizing the ambulatory surgery facilities. As noted in Table 12:1, 7,368 surgical procedures have been performed in the 1970-75 period; the majority were gynecological procedures. It should be noted,

however, that one of the criteria which we had for utilization of the ambulatory surgery service was that patients could not be operated on in the unit if they lived more than one hour away from the hospital. Because of this stipulation, there were approximately 1,800 additional urological patients who were hospitalized on a "24-hour admission" that could well have been operated on in the ambulatory surgery unit. Because of our favorable experience, we are currently revising this rule.

TABLE 12:1   NUMBER OF PATIENTS (1970-1975)

Gynecological (D&C, laparoscopies, V.T.P.)	3,858
Urological (Cystos, T.U.R.B., prostatic biopsy)	1,994
E.N.T. (Myringotomy, T&A)	217
Pain blocks	814
Miscellaneous (Plastics, orthopedic, general surgery)	563
TOTAL	7,368

2. *Age Distribution* (Table 12:2)—It should be noted that patients in all age groups have been operated on in the unit. In comparing these statistics with other ambulatory surgery units, there are a relatively small number of pediatric patients and a relatively small number of ENT patients. This is primarily due to the fact that in Seattle most of the pediatric surgery is performed in a children's hospital. Were this not the case, many more patients would have been operated on in the ambulatory surgery unit.

TABLE 12:2   AGE DISTRIBUTION

Age	No. of Patients
0-9	216
10-19	594
20-29	1,888
30-39	1,537
40-49	955
50-59	1,056
60-69	743
70-79	277
80-89	42
90-99	3

3. *Hospital Occupancy* (Table 12:3)—Many hospital administrators fear that an ambulatory surgery unit would merely shift inpatients to an outpatient status with a resultant decrease in hospital occupancy. Table 12:3 indicates that in spite of the fact that there was a steady increase in the number of short-stay surgical cases, the overall hospital occupancy did not change. The apparent dip in occupancy in 1970 was actually due to an addition of 35 beds in the hospital.

TABLE 12:3 HOSPITAL OCCUPANCY

Year	Occupancy	Total Surgical Cases	Short Stay Cases	Percent of Total Surgery
1968	89.2	6,039	—	—
1969	86.4	6,353	486	7.6
1970*	79.6	6,621	829	12.5
1971	75.9	7,363	1,448	19.7
1972	77.6	7,407	1,578	21.3
1973	79.7	7,911	1,795	22.7
1974	81.5	8,272	1,791	21.6

*Addition of 35 beds

4. *Type of Anesthesia* (Table 12:4)—Many different agents and techniques of anesthesia were used. None seemed to be superior either in awakening time, absence of nausea and vomiting, amnesia, or patient satisfaction. Most of the regional block procedures recorded were pain blocks.

TABLE 12:4 ANESTHETIC TECHNIQUES

Pentothal — N_2O — Halothane	982
Pentothal — N_2O	2,756
Brevital — N_2O	148
Pentothal — N_2O — relaxant	1,485
Pentothal — N_2O — narcotic	729
Regional block (exclusive pain blocks)	68
Miscellaneous (Cyclo, Penthrane, Ketamine)	211

5. *Time Spent in Unit* (Table 12:5)—The mean anesthesia time was approximately one hour and ten minutes and the mean surgery time was a little bit under an hour. It should be noted that the standard deviation

was considerable; this is primarily the result of the inclusion of a number of laparoscopic procedures some of which were very prolonged. One of the reasons advocated for a hospital-based ambulatory surgery unit is the necessity for hospital back-up for patient admissions. There were 71 patients scheduled for the ambulatory surgery unit who were admitted to the hospital postsurgery. Most of these were simply for patient convenience—i.e., they were sleepy after having late afternoon surgery; they were slightly nauseated; or they had just been looking forward to having a rest in the hospital. There were no patients in the series that had an emergency which could not be handled in the unit.

TABLE 12:5 TIME SPENT IN UNIT

Mean anesthesia time	69.66 minutes	S.D..±73.28
Mean surgery time	54.08 minutes	S.D.±56.99
Patients admitted	71	

6. *Type of Surgical Cases* (Table 12:6)—This table shows that the establishment of the short-stay surgery unit did not result in increased utilization for simple cases or in an increased number of inpatients which would increase the average length of hospital stay. The ratio of simple to complex cases remained approximately the same through the five years. The experience with the ambulatory surgery unit encouraged surgeons to also ambulate and discharge their more complex cases from the hospital sooner so that the length of stay of the average surgical patient actually decreased.

TABLE 12:6 TYPE OF SURGICAL CASES

Year	Simple	Complex	Length Of Stay
1968	2,724	3,315	6.9
1969	2,802	3,551	6.9
1970	2,716	3,908	6.6
1971	3,178	4,185	6.8
1972	2,828	4,579	7.0
1973	3,404	4,507	5.9
1974	3,420	4,852	6.0

7. *Dollars Saved Each Year* (Table 12:7)—These figures are calculated on the basis of the cost of a hospital room for one night and the admitting charges which would normally have been incurred by the short-stay service patients had they been admitted to the hospital.

TABLE 12:7   DOLLARS SAVED EACH YEAR

1968	—
1969	$ 27,200
1970	47,700
1971	87,600
1972	103,400
1973	118,500
1974	129,800

By 1974, utilization of the surgical suite was over 80% and the postanesthesia recovery unit was inadequate to handle the increased surgical volume. Consequently, additional recovery room space and additional operating rooms needed to be constructed. In planning and designing the construction for this additional space, the volume of ambulatory surgery was considered, and the newly constructed facilities were coordinated in order that the ambulatory surgery patients could be handled in a more convenient, personal, and expeditious manner. This was accomplished by constructing the new facilities immediately adjacent to the old operating suite and recovery room in the same manner as if it had been a newly constructed hospital-based satellite unit. The newly constructed space resulted in a new plan (Figure 12:1) which will rival a freestanding ambulatory surgery unit in convenience.

A review of the plan demonstrates how elective surgery for hospital inpatients (Flow Pattern A) is designed to operate immediately adjacent to the ambulatory surgery unit (Flow Pattern B). The plan offers flexibility of utilization of vacant operating rooms and unutilized personnel in either unit by the other service if the surgical volume of either is increased. The same applies to the contiguous postanesthesia recovery units. This plan offers the hospital flexibility for future expansion of either the inpatients or the ambulatory surgery volume if new anesthetics, new operations, or new federal standards should change the ratio of inpatient to ambulatory surgery patients without the construction of additional facilities.

As a result of our six years' experience with a hospital-based *integrated* ambulatory surgery unit, I am convinced that such a unit can provide facilities for the ambulatory surgery patient as conveniently and efficiently as a specialized freestanding or hospital satellite unit without additional cost resulting from duplicate construction costs for facilities or personnel. This assumes,

FIGURE 12:1   FLOW PATTERNS IN EXPANDED FACILITIES

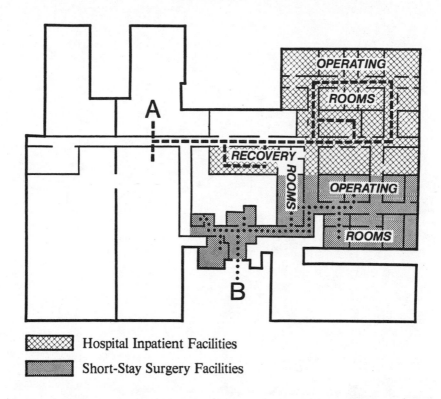

Hospital Inpatient Facilities

Short-Stay Surgery Facilities

however, that the hospital administrator recognizes that the ambulatory surgery service is a special service requiring individualization of admitting procedures; appropriate laboratory requirements; conveniently located waiting
room, interview, and dressing facilities; special operating room handling; and
special charges for all of these procedures. Personnel working in these areas as
well as in the necessary laboratory, operating room, and postanesthesia recovery rooms must be specially trained to understand ambulatory patients. The
success or failure of an ambulatory surgery unit is dependent much more on
the dedication and interest of the personnel than on the actual type of unit.

PART III
INDEPENDENTLY OPERATED
AMBULATORY SURGICAL CENTERS

Part III contains a complete description of the major issues and case studies relating to the freestanding independently operated ambulatory surgical facilities of the U.S. Leading the list is the famous landmark, award-winning program developed by Drs. Wallace A. Reed and John L. Ford, the Phoenix Surgicenter® of Phoenix, Arizona. The first chapter of Part III, by Wallace A. Reed, MD, presents a complete analysis of the Phoenix Surgicenter®. A special standard of health care delivery in ambulatory surgery has been put forth that our nation's hospitals may be hard-pressed to meet. Drs. Reed and Ford direct and manage a health care facility that provides dignity to the patient, efficiency and effectiveness in administration, and has a reputation as the finest independently operated health care facility in the U.S. today.

Another major case study of an independently operated facility was presented at the two most recent conferences of AAMA on ambulatory surgery by M. Robert Knapp, MD, cofounder of the Minor Surgery Center® of Wichita, in Wichita, Kansas. Dr. Knapp explains in full detail his philosophy is that the control of the patient should be returned to the physician for his input and direction. He is concerned about the bureaucracy of hospitals in the delivery of ambulatory surgery. In Chapter 13 Dr. Knapp presents a review of the Minor Surgery Center® of Wichita. One innovation of Dr. Knapp and his associates is transferring the patient to a "wake up" area rather than to a "recovery" area. Hospitals invariably use the term "recovery" area, which Dr. Knapp and his associates feel is inappropriate because the patients are not sick.

Jeffry C. Faine, administrator of the Ambulatory Surgical Facility, in Hollywood, Florida, provides a case study of the major activities of organization and other related issues. He stresses the importance of the freestanding independently operated surgical facilities and their role in the delivery of health care in the U.S. today. The chapter authored by Mr. Faine rounds out a fine description of the major contributions and organizational development of independently operated freestanding surgical facilities.

The concluding chapter in Part III was taken in large part from an article by the author which appeared in the Winter 1975 issue of *Hospital Administration*. This chapter presents some of the comparisons between the hospital ambulatory surgery facilities and the independently operated ambulatory surgery facilities. While there are major advantages to both approaches, there is no clear-cut conclusion that one system is superior to the other. Both have their place in the delivery of ambulatory surgical care.

Chapter 13
Taking Some Cobwebs Out of the Ambulatory Surgical Picture

Wallace A. Reed, MD

The objective of this chapter is to describe how a surgical facility for ambulatory patients was established. Such a facility can be established beneath the administrative umbrella of a hospital, but only if certain basic requirements are met. As for why we didn't develop our idea within the framework of the hospital, our experience in these matters leads us to believe that it would simply take too long.

Consider the climate in 1968 and 1969 when Dr. Ford, co-owner of the Surgicenter,® and I were studying the feasibility of establishing a surgical unit for ambulatory patients. Reviewing the literature, we found that Drs. Dillon and Cohen had published an article on the subject in *JAMA*.[1] They pointed out that the medical profession was being confronted by a bed shortage of indefinite duration, and urged giving attention to one-day stays for patients with certain surgical requirements. They reported on their experience during 1963 and 1964. During those two years, care was rendered to 1,523 patients (an average of about three patients per day), 47% under local anesthesia.

CONCLUSION NUMBER 1: "GEAR UP FOR POSSIBLE SHORTAGE OF HOSPITAL BEDS"

Drs. Charles Coakley and Marie-Louise Levy of George Washington University Hospital reported in 1967 that 2,114 cases had been performed in their in-and-out facility during the first year of operation.[2] Seven hundred fifty-eight of these were under general or regional anesthesia. Coakley and Levy experimented with the in-and-out concept because of crowded conditions in hospitals. They stressed the need to inform the insurance carriers of the savings they would enjoy under this type of program, a point also made by Dillon and Cohen.

CONCLUSION NUMBER 2:   LET'S IMPROVE THE ORGANIZATION AND DELIVERY OF AMBULATORY HEALTH CARE SERVICES.

In December of 1968 a National Advisory Commission on Health Facilities established by President Johnson gave its report. Commission Chairman Boisfeuillet Jones gave President Johnson several suggestions containing references to experimentation and efficiency and concluded with the observation that emphasis should be placed on improving the less developed components of comprehensive health care, such as the organization and delivery of ambulatory health care services.[3]

CONCLUSION NUMBER 3:   LET'S GET INSURANCE COVERAGE FOR OUTPATIENTS

Also in 1968, Dr. Dwight Wilbur, President of the American Medical Association, stressed the following points in several talks.[4]

- As doctors, we need to assume responsibility for the costs of medical care and to increase our concern for expenditure for hospital care.
- We must try to hold down patients' expenditures by making use of hospitals only when clearly necessary.
- We should continue our efforts to achieve wider insurance and prepayment coverage outside of the hospital.

Here again is the challenge to focus on outpatient care, eliminate unnecessary hospitalization, and broaden insurance benefits.

In November of 1969 Blue Cross Association President Walter McNerney called for cutting red tape in billing and for giving hospitals more incentives to cut costs.[5] While the Surgicenter's® ultimate service to the community will be to reduce the time people must wait to have elective operations, we have meanwhile demonstrated a certain capacity for giving hospitals incentives to cut costs. Charges to patients for ambulatory surgical procedures have been reduced in seven Phoenix area hospitals since the opening of the Surgicenter® three years ago. Our prompt and effective response to McNerney's request was inadvertent. We did not see ourselves in a competitive role with hospitals. We see ourselves as taking over a chore which hospitals seemed unwilling or unprepared to assume. Although hospitals had all the advantages, including a 60-year head-start, they didn't advance the concept of ambulatory surgery.

McNerney further stated in December 1969 that in order to keep health care costs within reason, the incentive for a patient to occupy a costly hospital bed should be reduced. About the same time, Dr. William Dornette, an authority on the subject, gave a paper entitled, "Planning Tomorrow's Hospital Today." In this paper, Dr. Dornette stated: "One facility about which little has been written is the outpatient service offering general anesthesia for minor surgical procedures. The operation of one such facility as part of a hospital's outpatient department, and the advantages accrued to such operation, are well documented. But a safe and efficient facility for the performance of general anesthesia and minor surgical procedures need not be affiliated either administratively or geographically with a hospital''.[7]

Here then, were the President of the AMA, the President of Blue Cross Association and the Chairman of a Presidential Commission—along with many others—calling for experimentation in health care delivery, for lower utilization of hospital beds, and for emphasis on outpatient care. Practical medical practitioners, such as Dr. Dillon at UCLA and Dr. Coakley at George Washington University Hospital, were showing us how it could be done with surgical cases, and Dr. Dornette was pointing out that such a facility need not be affiliated either administratively or geographically with a hospital.

To Dr. Ford and myself, this was a challenge to which we simply had to respond. Although we were convinced our idea to establish an independent facility was sound, it wasn't easy to convince others. At the outset, we were naive enough to think that government and industry might be willing to give us some financial help. But we soon learned the Little Red Hen's lesson: When we asked, "Who will help us build?" we heard, "Not I," from the Department of Health, Education, and Welfare. "Not I," from industry and labor. So we did it ourselves. With the help of a nurse, we worked out a design for the operating and recovery rooms and traffic flow through these rooms. With a local bank, we also worked out arrangements for financing. No government funds were involved.

We obtained approval from the Comprehensive Health Planning Council of Maricopa County, the County Medical Society, and the State Medical Association. With the help of these groups, we worked out suitable methods of quality control. We provided information on our intentions to everyone who asked, keeping the following people and organizations informed: the administrators of three local hospitals; the AMA; the American Board of Anesthesiology; the Academy of Anesthesiology; the American Society of Anesthesiologists; the Arizona Health Planning Authority; the Arizona Department of Health; and various state legislators and national senators and congressmen.

Looking at the track record, we have completed over 13,000 cases. Some tables were made at the 9,000 point, but are representative of over 30,000 cases now. These tables are now presented. They will provide the reader with a good overview of the basic picture of our Surgicenter's® major activity in our early years.

TABLE 13:1   MOST OFTEN PERFORMED PROCEDURES
(OF 9,000 CASES)

Diagnostic D&C (no therapeutics are performed)	1,734
Myringotomy	573
Inguinal Herniorrhaphy	542
Excision of Skin Lesion	498
Vasectomy	338
Laparoscopy	245
Ganglionectomy	242
Adenoidectomy	240
Cystoscopy	219
Circumcision	133
Tonsillectomy	126
Eye Muscle Operation	121
Other	3,988

TABLE 13:2   MOST COMMONLY PERFORMED PROCEDURES
(SERIES OF 33,000)

Diagnostic D & C	6,311
Laparoscopy	4,332
Myringotomies	1,633
Inguinal Herniorrhaphies	1,607
Adenoidectomy	1,407
Excision Skin Lesions	1,069
Excision Ganglion	725
Vasectomy	630
Cystoscopy	528
Eye Muscle	514
Other	14,244
Total	33,000

TABLE 13:3   CASES ACCORDING TO SPECIALTY
(OF 9,000)

Gynecology	2,506
General Surgery	1,996
ENT	1,325
Orthopedic	1,210
G-U	1,008
Plastic	440
Eye	306
Dental	56
Other	153

TABLE 13:4   CLASSIFICATION ACCORDING TO AGE

Under 2 Years	8.69%
Between 2 and 65	88.56%
Over 65	2.75%

TABLE 13:5   DAILY AVERAGE NUMBER OF PATIENTS

First Year	12
Second Year	16
Third Year	20
Fourth Year (projected)	28

TABLE 13:6   NUMBER OF CASES PER YEAR

First Year	2,528
Second Year	4,046
Third Year	5,116
Fourth Year (projected)	7,160

TABLE 13:7   PERSONNEL NEEDED   (EXCLUSIVE OF PHYSICIANS) FOR 500-550 CASES PER MONTH

Medical	16
Clerical	10
Other	3

REGISTERED NURSES

Operating Room	10
PAR	6*

OTHER

Instrument Tech	1
Maintenance Tech (Medical)	2

*One of these rotates as needed in OR.

TABLE 13:8   CLERICAL

Admitting Scheduling Secretary	2
Account Clerks	4
Receptionist-Typist	1
Medical Transciptionist	1
Housekeeping/Maintenance	1
Office Manager	1
Total	10

This makes a total of 29 employees, or an employee-patient relationship of 1:1.

TABLE 13:9   COST COMPARISONS FOR THE PHOENIX AREA
(1973)

Cost of eye recession, bilateral, at a local hospital, total of 21 itemized charges, $456 (including SMA 12, Triglycerides and pulmonary screening on a healthy youngster)

Cost at Surgicenter®	$168.00
Difference	288.00
Laparoscopy and Tubal Coagulation	
Hospital Inpatient	332.00
Hospital Outpatient	236.00
Surgicenter®	144.00
Savings vs. Inpatient	188.00
Savings vs. Outpatient	92.00

CONCLUSION

Many people who have visited us (and there have been over a thousand) think the Surgicenter's® secret is that it is a building situated apart from a hospital. In Phoenix, there are two administrators who have built such facilities, thereby admitting—as we have claimed from the beginning—that they believe present-day hospitals are not designed to accommodate the ambulatory surgical patient. We may soon learn if the changed location does anything new for the hospital's ambulatory surgical service. These two new facilities are under the administrative umbrella of the hospital, and are, therefore, simply extensions of the already existing outpatient department.

In the opinion of Dr. Ford and myself, the improvement will not be brought about simply by changing the location of the outpatient unit. The answer lies in the ability to respond to a deeply felt community need: Essentially, what we have recognized and acted on at the Surgicenter® is that people like to be treated like people. They like to be talked to and not down to. They like to know in advance what their service is to cost them. They like to have a sense of identity, and a sense of autonomy. They want a sense of control over their environment.

At the Surgicenter,® these desires are satisfied, both for patients and personnel. The patients are treated like people, and as equals. We regard them as responsible individuals who want to get well and try to get well; persons who follow instructions. Because we treat them with respect and expect them to act in their own best interests, they respond accordingly.

An illustration may be helpful here. At the hospital when patients become nauseated postop, they ask that something be done for them or given to them. Their appeal is to ask the doctor to help them. At the Surgicenter® patients' responses are moie likely to be to assure the doctor that they are feeling better all the time, and will be fine as soon as they go home. This confirms the finding we see daily of Wilson et al. that one of the major desires of most patients in all age groups is to go home as soon as possible after an operation.[8]

We also treat children like people. The fact they too are individuals is sometimes overlooked in hospitals. At the Surgicenter®, all of our activities—except the actual surgical procedure—are carried out under the watchful eyes of the parents. In the pediatric room the parents stay with the unpremedicated child until it is time for him to be taken to the operating room. Here, in the pediatric room, the child is often delivered from the arms of the parent to the arms of the OR nurse—a moment when extreme tact and evidence of concern are called for. It is both amazing and rewarding to observe this transfer accomplished almost always without upsetting the child's (or the parents') emotional balance.

There is another principle we follow at Surgicenter®. It is as difficult for doctors to understand about administrators as it is for administrators to understand about doctors. Doctors are also people; we like to have our suggestions taken seriously and not smothered in a mass of red tape. We find no satisfaction in making suggestions which fall on deaf ears. When a doctor makes a request for a certain type of suture or prep solution, he doesn't like an OR nurse to tell him that he can take his patients somewhere else, if he doesn't like it there.

We believe nurses are people, too, and they are too-often neglected. We consulted them during the formative stages. We still consult them, and many of their ideas are incorporated both in the bricks and mortar and in the concept. Little time is lost in giving substance to ideas which seem worthwhile. Their suggestions, as well as the suggestions of surgeons using the facility, are given the serious attention they deserve. Other personnel are also considered important: receptionists, secretaries, bookkeepers, telephone operators, insurance clerks, and maintenance men are made to feel they are an integral part of the Surgicenter® team.

We found it extremely helpful in treating people with respect for another reason. In doing so, we tapped a valuable source of paramedical help in the form of parents, relatives, and friends of patients. They are responsible people, who, when given the opportunity, respond eagerly to help a patient who is close to them. They have made a significant contribution in helping us achieve our objectives.

In response to the challenges we defined previously, our objectives are:
- To elevate the status of the ambulatory patient's surgical care.
- To streamline the delivery of surgical services.
- To reduce the cost of care.
- To work for a broadening of insurance coverage.
- To accomplish these objectives in an environment that is pleasant for patients, office personnel, doctors, and nurses to work in.

We think we are well on the way to accomplishing these objectives.

Can this environment be duplicated within the administrative framework of the hospital? I think it can if (1) you decentralize your operation so as to develop a person-centered organization; (2) you create a situation where individuals have an enhanced self-concept and sense of control over their environment; and (3) within the framework of your hospital, you can accord ambulatory patients the individualized treatment and quality care they want, expect, and deserve.

Can your hospitals meet these challenges?

Notes

1. David D. Cohen and John B. Dillon, "Anesthesia for Outpatient Surgery," *JAMA*, Vol. 196, 1966, p. 1114.

2. Charles S. Coakley and Marie-Louise Levy, "Anesthesia for Ambulatory Surgery." (Paper presented at Annual Meeting of the Arkansas Medical Society, Hot Springs, Arkansas, April 26-27, 1971.)

3. Boisfeuillet Jones, Chairman, National Advisory Commission on Health Facilities, as reported in *AMA News*, December 23, 1968.

4. Dwight L. Wilbur, M.D., "Let's Lead Rather Than Be Led," a paper read before the New England Postgraduate Assembly, Boston, November 6, 1968.

5. Walter J. McNerney, "How to Improve Medical Care," *U.S. News and World Report*, March 24, 1969, p. 42.

6. The "Surgicenter" name is registered and legally protected to refer only to the Surgicenter, 1040 East McDowell Road, Phoenix, Arizona 85006.

7. William H. L. Dornette, M.D., "Planning Tomorrow's Hospital Today," (Paper given at the A.S.A. meeting in Washington, Oct. 1968.)

8. E. Wilson, "Preoperative Anxiety and Anesthesia: Their Relation," *Anesthesia and Analgesia* Vol. 48, 1969, pp. 605-611.

Chapter 14
The Return of Control of the Patient to the Physician

M. Robert Knapp, MD

The primary objective in developing a freestanding surgical facility should be to meet the community's needs. The hospital in the contemplated area of a freestanding surgical facility should regard it as a unit which is complimentary to hospital goals, functioning for the betterment of the hospital, physicians, community and, most of all, the patient. The hospital industry of the City of Wichita did not regard the Minor Surgery Center of Wichita as being complimentary to its goals. Rather, the development of our freestanding ambulatory surgical facility was strewn with many obstacles.

The genesis of the freestanding ambulatory surgical facility is the private practitioner's response to the high cost of medical care. Facilities, such as my own, appear to be an appropriate response to this challenge. We are rendering high quality surgical care at lower cost to the patient.

There is no question that with the astronomical rise of hospital costs, the federal government, the provider of over 40% of the health care dollar, will do something about containing these costs if it is not done by the free enterprise system. A natural response is to take minor surgical procedures out of the hospital environment into an environment like a freestanding ambulatory surgical facility. In such a facility minor surgery costs are not prohibitive, and the patient pays only for what he is getting. The doctor can once more resume complete control of his patient. By their inefficient use of professional time and patient inconvenience, hospitals do drive up the dollar expense to the patient, or to the third party payer responsible for such payment. The patient for minor surgery need not be hospitalized in elaborate facilities. The highly sophisticated services the hospital can provide are unnecessary for such patients. It has been estimated that upwards of fifteen billion dollars could be saved annually in health care costs, if all minor surgical procedures were done on an outpatient basis. These costs must necessarily be a substantial element in the total health care costs experienced by any community.

123

In certain areas of the U.S., where operating room space is not available for the surgical patient, the cost to the public may be measured in terms of delayed treatment for all patients, which in turn means a lower than acceptable quality of medical care in that particular community.

Because of their small size and very limited function, freestanding ambulatory surgical facilities will always be able to deliver better service at a lower cost than larger health care institutions. We believe that by providing specialized facilities for minor surgical procedures, Minor Surgery Center,® and other similar facilities, are making it possible for hospitals to concentrate on the major cases, which actually require hospitalization. From the perspective of cost accounting, there is no justification for the patient receiving minor surgical care to pay for the cost of expensive equipment, facilities or personnel when he does not use them. The patient who uses these services should pay for them. By the same token, it is wasteful to expand existing hospital bed space when the need for such additional capacity might well be avoided or reduced through the construction of minor surgical facilities at a fraction of the cost.

The goal of Minor Surgery Center® and all other freestanding surgical facilities is to provide the physician and the patient with an environment where the work can be done with a minimum amount of interference, delay or distractions. Minor Surgery Center® is simply an extension of the physician's own office; it has instituted only those regulations which are necessary to record the events which occur in the institution itself. It seeks to maximize the time during which the physician can concentrate directly upon the needs of his patient.

Even though the hospitals attempt to improve ambulatory surgical care by remodeling or even segregating the facilities which they maintain for this purpose, the contrast with Minor Surgery Center® is remarkable. First the patient no longer has to tolerate cancellation of his surgery due to a large number of unanticipated major cases. Such cancellations, or the possibility of them occurring, are a source of anxiety for every minor surgical patient, even before reaching the hospital. Minor Surgery Center,® as well as other freestanding ambulatory surgical facilities, always provides an operating room at the time scheduled. Scheduling, admission and release of the patient are all greatly simplified in these facilities. Just as important as the patient's peace of mind, is the surgeon's confidence that he can do the procedure when it is scheduled. The savings are substantial because of his increased efficiency, and even more importantly, he can concentrate entirely upon the requirements of his patients. Both are relaxed and better prepared for the operation.

Even if the hospital ambulatory surgical facility is entirely detached and segregated from the hospital itself, rotating personnel, complex admission requirements and other difficulties associated with larger institutions may still remain. These are the very factors which have increased both the cost of health care and the anxiety associated with hospitalization.

Since ambulatory surgical facilities are primarily designed to enhance the patient-physician relationship, and to provide simple support services, Minor Surgery Center® believes that physicians are particularly well qualified to own and operate minor surgery facilities. They, more than any group, are familiar with the needs of doctors and patients. This critical factor is the most difficult to regulate. Within the community of physicians who would otherwise be qualified to operate ambulatory surgical facilities, anesthesiologists have the advantage of being unable to refer patients to such facilities—surgeons make such decisions in consultation with their patients. Thus, a conflict of interest is avoided.

The advantage inherent in freestanding ambulatory surgical facilities is that they constitute an effective alternative to a conventional mode of patient care. Such facilities will serve the dual purpose: holding down the cost of similar procedures performed at hospitals; and providing a partial solution for the congested surgical suites in our major hospitals. It is difficult to imagine a more effective way in which to simultaneously reduce costs and improve the quality of health care delivery to U.S. citizens. These reasons explain the enthusiastic endorsement of such facilities by the General Accounting Office in the report entitled, "Study of Health Facilities Construction Costs," published in October 1972.

Freestanding ambulatory surgical facilities are directly responsible to the physicians and patients who utilize them. Regardless of the location of the facility it will only be successful if it satisfies both physicians and patients. If the facility is successful, its stockholders will earn a fair return on their investment. Freestanding ambulatory surgical facilities should be permitted to take the risk of their own success or failure since the health care delivery system in this country can only benefit as a result.

Outpatient surgery without overnight hospitalization is not a new concept. The first research study performed was reported in a paper presented at a meeting of the British Medical Association in 1909, by Dr. J. H. Nichol of Glasgow. He reported on 7,323 operations which he had performed on ambulatory patients at the Royal Glasgow Hospital for Children. Advantages were reported for both the patient and the family. Since that time the popularity of surgical outpatient procedures has varied depending upon the community, the public and the physician.

The main reason for the success of Minor Surgery Center® is that the patient is the primary concern. Since the entire organization is patient oriented, the patient encounters only those people who are directly involved in his care. The orientation is immediately obvious to the patient the moment he enters the center. The patient's first encounter with the nurse is pleasant and reassuring. Laboratory work and directions to the patient and his family regarding his procedure are given carefully and quickly. Our nurses are encouraged to study each patient and, if possible, to establish his fears and seek to allay them. All questions are answered courteously and promptly. The laboratory work at the center is to determine if the patient is an adequate anesthetic risk. This involves a routine urinalysis and hemoglobin. The patient's temperature, blood pressure and weight are recorded. These tests, together with the anesthesiologist's history and physical examination, provide an adequate basis for determining the physical status of the patient.

The anesthesiologist responsible for administering the anesthetic sees the patient soon after his arrival. This interview is brief, thorough and, above all, reassuring to the patient. The anesthesiologist examines the patient's heart and lungs and reassures the patient concerning his care at the center. During this interview and examination the patient may ask questions, and every effort is made to answer them thoroughly and completely. The patient is then seen by the surgeon before being taken to the operating room.

The circulating nurse in charge of the operating room introduces herself to the patient and assures the patient that she will be with him in the operating room during the entire procedure. The nurse will personally take the patient to the operating room on the operating room cart and help the patient to transfer to the operating room table. All the nursing personnel in the operating room are chosen for their warm personalities and efficiency in surgical nursing. The nurse's first contact with the patient is warm, friendly and reassuring. As the patient enters the operating room, the anesthesiologist again greets him and reassures him.

Following the surgical procedure, the patient is transferred to the recovery room. It should be noted that the surgeon's only contact with the patient at Minor Surgery Center® has been the greeting and performance of the surgical procedure. The surgeon is not involved with the preoperative examination, admitting procedures or chart work. The surgeon performs the operation, immediately dictates the procedure while still in the operating room, and signs the chart as surgeon. He writes any specific postoperative orders and leaves the building. Postoperative care, dismissal of the patient and further chart work is performed by the anesthesiologist.

The anesthesiologist will see the patient again in the recovery room area and will dismiss the patient from the Minor Surgery Center® after he is certain that all is well. The attendance of the anesthesiologist in the recovery room is an important factor in outpatient surgical care. Every effort is made to assure the patient that his well-being after leaving the center is of major interest to the center. Directions are given to tell him what to expect during the remainder of the day while recuperating at home. The anesthesiologist is readily available for consultation with the nurse in the recovery room if necessary. The operating rooms are only a few steps away from the recovery room area. If necessary, the patient can be returned to the operating room area for care. As soon as the patient is receptive, he is encouraged to take liquid nourishment in the form of soft drinks, coffee, tea or soups. Children are also encouraged to take liquids. We find, however, that children are delighted with eating popsicles, so we keep a large supply on hand.

The pediatric recovery procedures are somewhat different from those of adults in that the immediate family is utilized as paramedical personnel. A member of the family is encouraged to be at the child's bedside as soon as vital signs are stable. This means that the child's first encounter postoperatively is with a familiar face, a familiar touch, and a familiar voice. This presence is not only helpful to the patient but to the parent as well. No patient who receives general anesthesia is allowed to leave the Minor Surgery Center® under his own guidance. All patients must be accompanied by a friend or relative.

Part of the success of the center concept comes from the surgeon's convenience in caring for patients. The surgeon does what he is supposed to do: perform surgery and sign as the responsible agent. This aspect is greatly appreciated by the surgeon; it differs considerably from the usual hospital procedures.

The construction of any ambulatory surgical facility should not be undertaken without the concurrence of the local medical community. In the case of the Minor Surgery Center,® the support of the local County Medical Society was solicited and obtained. All quality control of the surgical events within the center resides in the local county medical society through its appointed Surgical Advisory Committee. Thus, we believe that we have effectively returned *the control of the patient to the doctor*. There is no intervention of administration or nursing service in this very important patient-physician relationship. The fact that the facility is owned and operated by physicians makes it much easier for it to be responsive to the wishes of the medical staff as well as the patient. For this reason, harmonious relationships which exist among the patient, nurse and physician have been a source of constant reassurance to those of us involved in this effort. Many patients who come here now, do so because a friend or casual acquaintance has been a patient at the center. That patient enthusiastically recounted his experience to the friend who requests admission to the center by his surgeon. A slogan which summarizes the methodology of the center might well be, "maximizing patient care, minimizing paper work."

Surgical facilities contain all the medications and equipment needed for operations that are expected to be performed. We also have provisions for the physical and emotional well-being of our patients and their relatives as well as those services necessary for any emergencies which may arise within the facility. We have also designed an efficient administrative system providing easy access to medical records, statistical data and efficient storage of this information. In the construction of the center, which is licensed by the State of Kansas, we have met all applicable local and state fire, safety, sanitation, and building codes. We have adopted procedures to minimize the sources and transmission of infection within the unit. We have developed a bacteriological surveillance method based on frequent cultures of all areas of the Minor Surgery Center.® All combustible materials and supplies are handled in such a manner as to minimize the chance of fire. All this handling is done in conformance with local fire safety codes and regulations. Those drugs which are utilized within the facility are stored and dispensed properly and refrigerated if deemed necessary. Drugs requiring refrigeration are stored in their own separate refrigerator. All drug supplies are constantly monitored to replace those items which have become outdated. All outdated items are promptly discarded. The Minor Surgery Center® has a complement of fire extinguishers, all of which are approved by Underwriter Laboratories, which are inspected and tagged annually to make sure that they have not been tampered with, or removed from their designated places. These extinguishers are checked periodically for defects or content change.

The admittance of patients' personnel and visitors to our operating room is constantly monitored and controlled. No surgical procedure is undertaken at Minor Surgery Center® unless we have the proper equipment and personnel to do such a procedure. It must be emphasized that the medical staff and the Surgical Advisory Committee are in constant contact with the daily schedule at the center, providing the adequate supervision and control necessary to insure high quality surgical care. Following the completion of the operation, when the surgeon has dictated the procedure, the dictation is transcribed by a medical secretary to the permanent records. This accurate, complete description of the findings and technique of surgery is generally completed within twenty-four hours of the surgical procedures. All tissues removed in surgery are sent to a pathologist of the surgeon's choice. At the Minor Surgery Center,® the surgeon makes a decision as to what tissue will be sent to which pathologist. This negates the need for the sending of such obvious things as toenails, teeth, and hardware to the pathologist for expensive laboratory examination. Documentation of removal is evident within the center's record. Minor Surgery Center® has the capacity to get blood or blood products to its patients, if needed (since our opening date, there has been no need for this type of therapy). The most modern type of resuscitation and suction equipment is available for our patients at all times.

All equipment within the center receives constant preventive maintenance. This is a crucial aspect of outpatient surgical care. All equipment must be in good working condition in order to insure the safety of our patients. Equipment necessary for the administration of anesthetics is kept particularly clean. Electrical systems, vacuum systems, fire detection and smoke detection systems, endoscopes of various kinds, light sources, fiberoptic light carriers, the operating microscope and its component parts and the x-ray equipment must be checked regularly in order that they function perfectly.

The keystone in the arch of all ambulatory surgical facilities is the anesthesiologist. His attendance within the unit is absolutely essential for the smooth operation of such institutions. The anesthesiologist should be on the premises prior to the commencement of the first surgical case of the day, and should be in attendance throughout the entire day until the last patient has successfully left the facility.

Finally, the Minor Surgery Center® has proved to be an asset to the Wichita community. It has successfully bridged the gap existing between the physician's office and the hospital. Our unit does procedures that are too small for the hospital and too large for the office. The center was designed to provide minor surgery care to patients of all ages. In this regard, it is to be thought of as a specialty center for attention given to the infant, as well as the aged. The patient has assurance that his health insuror will provide him with coverage for this service. The surgeon has the assurance of ready convenience with minimal paper work. The community has the advantage of another health care facility which will be available to it in emergencies or disasters. The Minor Surgery Center® has responded to the challenge for the medical profession to reduce costs while maintaining quality care. It was our intention to do so when we began, and we believe that we have succeeded.

Chapter 15
The Position of Independently Operated Facilities

Jeffry C. Faine

Major health changes are taking place to elevate the level of patient care and to reduce or maintain the cost of health care delivery. One of the major changes is the recent innovation of same-day surgery centers. This discussion will focus on the freestanding ambulatory surgical hospital facilities.

An ambulatory surgical hospital facility shall be defined as a hospital facility for elective surgery, in which a patient walks in before the procedure, and walks out after—within the same working day. These are procedures that have customarily been done on an inpatient basis, though they can be done routinely on a same-day basis. Such a facility includes all elements to permit surgery, anesthesia, recovery and emergency measures, and meets all hospital standards, with the exception of maintaining overnight accommodations. The purpose of these facilities is to provide sophisticated surgical care within easy access of the patient, at less cost than similar services in a hospital.

The advantages of the ambulatory surgical facility are numerous:

1. Reduction of psychological trauma—both the child and adult will be returned to familiar surroundings (to their family and homes) the same day.
2. Recuperation occurs at home, where all people feel more comfortable.
3. Decreased period of disability.
4. Reduction of cross-infection.
5. Reduction of postoperative medication (narcotics only prolong recovery).
6. More personalized care.
7. Fast scheduling.
8. More effective use of physician time.
9. Reduction of unnecessary lab and x-ray tests.
10. More room for hospitals to handle the more seriously ill patients.
11. Reducing the need to construct new beds, or at least, reducing the number of beds needed.

12. Patient is able to return to work sooner.
13. A significant decrease in the expense of surgery for the patient, insurance company, the community and the government.

The ambulatory surgical hospital facility should have full disclosure of ownership and control. There shall be an organized governing body. This body shall have the ultimate responsibility and authority for conduct of the institution. The governing body shall adopt by-laws, identifying the purpose of the ambulatory surgical hospital facility. The governing body has the overall authority and responsibility for the conduct of the facility and making available high quality patient care. The governing body shall establish policies to insure that only members of the medical staff admit patients to the facility and that a physician member of the medical staff is responsible for the aspects of patient care. There shall be a formal organization of the medical staff, with formalized by-laws, and the overall authority for quality of medical care.

All ambulatory surgical hospital facilities shall be licensed by their appropriate State when licensure becomes available. They should apply at the earliest possible time and be accredited by the Joint Commission on Accreditation of Hospitals (JCAH) when regulations are adopted. These facilities shall maintain a written transfer agreement with one or more accredited hospitals.

The medical staff organization shall strive to create and maintain an optimum level of professional performance of its members through the appointment procedure, the delineation of medical staff privileges and the continued review and evaluation of each member's clinical activities. This continual review shall be established through medical audit, tissue committee, utilization, medical records and credentials committees. These committees shall meet periodically and review medical records, privileges, JCAH standards, medical operation of the facility, procedures capable of being performed and methods of determining new procedures to be performed. The ambulatory surgical hospital facility shall be used only for the purpose of performing surgical procedures that have been deemed suitable for ambulatory surgery by the governing authority on recommendation of the Medical Review Committee.

The ambulatory surgical hospital facility shall be sufficiently staffed and supervised at all times by adequately trained and experienced personnel. A board certified anesthesiologist shall be present for all procedures requiring anesthesia, and at all times when patients are in the facility. In the area of nursing services, the operating room, postoperative recovery room and patient observation areas shall have full-time supervision by registered professional nurses in accordance with JCAH standards.

Ambulatory surgical hospital facilities should be operated in a cost efficient manner which is responsive to identified health needs. Resources must be utilized so as to obtain the greatest impact on improving the health of the entire community. The ambulatory surgical services should be incorporated whenever possible into comprehensive health care programs, and in order to minimize duplication of services, the objectives and plans of such facilities should be coordinated with those of other health services in the community.

In assessing quality care, the Utilization Review Committee shall evaluate the appropriateness of admissions to the ambulatory surgical hospital facility, the length of patient stay, discharge and transfer practices, services to be rendered, and all other related factors which may contribute to effective utilization of the facility. In further assessing the quality of patient care in such facilities, one finds that less than one-half of a percent of the patients treated have been referred to acute hospitals for further care. Also, the current infection rate in these facilities is less than one-half of a percent. This is considerably below the acute hospitals. Fear of possible complications has been studied, both in the United States and England. The results indicate that complications will be apparent before the patient is discharged from the facility, so that proper follow-up care can be started. One final assessment of quality care is the fact that ambulatory facilities have proved that they have been able to return patients to productive members of society quicker than existing acute hospital facilities.

Today, inpatient hospital services consume more than half of the nation's health care expenditures. Ambulatory surgical hospital facilities are making a significant impact in reducing and controlling health care expenditures. Studies have been conducted across the nation which show such savings. In 1971, a Duke University Hospital study showed a dollar savings of 25% and a savings of over two patient days. Similar studies conducted in Milwaukee, Washington D.C., Phoenix, Hollywood (Florida), Wichita and Los Angeles have shown savings from 25-60% and bed saving utilization between two and three days.

It has been estimated that 20-40% of all surgical procedures can be performed on a same-day basis. The Professional Hospital Activities Study lists five procedures which constitute 25% of all surgical volume. These procedures are: diagnostic D&C, T&A, skin procedures, hemorrhoids and diagnostic cystoscopies; and they are currently being performed daily in all of the same-day facilities. If we accept the conservative amount of 25%, an estimated reduction in health care expenditures will be in excess of $350 million. Further savings are seen by the economy of time savings to the surgeon, who can see more patients and utilize his time more appropriately for patients with greater need. In addition to the economy of physicians' time, we see better utilization of paramedical personnel, many of whom perform mulitple tasks and jobs, thus reducing the payroll.

It is estimated that approximately 25-33% of all surgery appropriate for ambulatory surgical facilities would save billions of dollars a year.

Today it is evident that the demands placed on the modern acute hospital are rapidly making the cost of elective surgery prohibitive. Included here are: inefficient use of professional time and patient inconvenience, need for special arrangements, loss of work, and having the life style and schedule of the family disturbed during the hospital admission. Much of the cost is related directly to the fact that many patients are hospitalized in elaborate facilities, when they do not need the highly sophisticated services of a modern acute hospital. Their presence in a hospital in turn imposes a serious burden on those patients who actually need the full resources of the acute hospital. Hospital admissions for elective surgery result in unnecessary charges for rooms and other services, and in many cases extra screening tests because the patient is in the hospital. These hospital costs and the costs of inefficiently utilized professional care and patient time become a significant element in health care costs to the community.

The long range impact of ambulatory surgical hospital facilities is measurable in real dollar savings and better utilization of existing hospital beds. Currently, it costs between $50,000 and $60,000 to build and equip one single hospital bed. If we drop the 20-40% of patients who qualify for same-day surgery from the hospital planning, we will have to build fewer beds in the future. A clear and absolute saving to the public will result. The bed days saved by Phoenix, Wichita and Hollywood, Florida facilities will be in excess of 90,000 patient days by the end of 1975. Comparable to a 500-bed acute general hospital, what would it cost to build such a facility? Current data has shown where ambulatory surgical hospital facilities have provided a definite reduction in construction cost and increased stability of beds for more acute patients. There has been only a slight effect on the surgical census in the existing hospitals. In fact, many hospitals have shown an increase and a more efficient use of the operating suites for the more acute type of surgical case. With National Health Insurance around the corner, the bed savings provided by ambulatory surgical hospital facilities will provide a real savings to the community in meeting the anticipated future demands.

It is the ultimate goal to develop a uniform cost, reimbursement, and utilization reporting system to improve management for health care institutions. A design of a uniform standard cost system that will reflect the cost charge relationship for every purchaser of health care is being developed at the Ambulatory Surgical Facility in Hollywood, Florida. This system will be designed to match revenues with cost, establishing a preliminary rate which is sensitive to competitive prices. It also will relate each procedure cost to known factors which reflect the quality of care and the cost of care rendered to the health care consumer. This system, if properly implemented, would save thousands of dollars for the health care consumer, would render better quality care at less cost, and yield cost benefits to the health care community. Further, the ambulatory surgical facility of Hollywood has already developed a daily charge audit, so that all charges billed have actually been performed and can be verified from the medical record. This will allow for an efficient and accurate billing system without undue overcharges or undercharges, providing significant savings in the efficient handling of all hospital charges. These are some of the real advantages in cost savings that ambulatory surgical hospital facilities on a freestanding basis can provide in the delivery of health care.

Ambulatory surgical hospital facilities can also make a significant contribution to cost reduction of the Medicare program. On a national basis, experience has shown that persons 65 years of age and over, as a group, require hospitalization more often and for longer stays. Persons in this age group comprise approximately 25% of hospital census days. Further, in the south Florida area these individuals comprise 60-70% of the hospital census days. Many of these individuals can have, and want to have, surgery on a same-day basis. But the current regulations force these individuals to an acute hospital where they stay too long and have unnecessary tests, thus escalating costs. In the south Florida area, the savings will be in the millions of dollars.

The government can encourage the use of ambulatory surgical hospital facilities: (1) by a reimbursement formula which would encourage same day surgery through coverage under governmental insurance programs; and (2) by imposing restrictions on the performance of inpatient surgery for those conditions which could as easily be performed in an ambulatory surgical facility. One hopes that we never have to reach the method of imposing restrictions.

In summary, ambulatory surgical hospital facilities provide more personal attention to the patients, better utilization of physician time, reduction of psychological trauma, faster scheduling, pre-and postoperative support by the family in a familiar situation, reduction of patients' time away from home, and faster return to work. We have also seen a reduction of the cross-infection rate. Further, this concept is providing direct and indirect cost savings to the patient and to the community with better utilization and more efficient use of costly components of the health care delivery system. In conclusion, we should make every effort to extend this concept to the nation as a whole.

Chapter 16
Hospitals Versus the Independents: Components of the Fight*

Thomas R. O'Donovan

A controversy is stirring and the stakes are high. Ambulatory surgery has now become a major market, and both hospitals and independent facilities are challenging one another in some sections of the country for these patients. Hospitals haven't always done a very good job, and over 60% of them do not even have a program of ambulatory surgery. Many patients may not be ready for short-stay surgery when hospitalization insurance pays for the inpatient costs. Are surgeons supportive of the short-stay surgery concept? Increasingly, the answer to this question is yes. Yet, thousands of patients spend one to three days in hospitals for procedures for which they could come-and-go on the same day.

As hospitals drop the ball, the independently operated surgical facilities are ready to take over and make a profit doing so.

The independently operated facilities list quite a barrage of "hospital problems of tradition" such as (1) long and impersonal admitting procedures; (2) delay in lab tests; (3) unpredictable surgical schedules; and (4) surgical patients in outpatient departments are generally regarded as second-class citizens. The independents also argue that the reason hospital charges for short surgical procedures are so high is that these patients help underwrite open heart surgery and other sophisticated procedures.

The key question now becomes, "Who *should* do it—the hospital or the independents?" Battle lines are being drawn. Many other questions need to be answered. What are the differences in costs of short-stay surgery among independents and hospitals? What about red tape, patient satisfaction, and community acceptance? (See Appendix B.)

Many independently operated surgical centers avidly claim that competition

---

*Parts of this chapter are adapted from Thomas R. O'Donovan, "Dynamics of Ambulatory Surgery," *Hospital and Health Services Administration*, pp. 27-39. Reprinted with permission from the quarterly journal of the American College of Hospital Administrators, *Hospital and Health Services Administration*, Winter, 1975.

is good for our nation's health care delivery system. Dr. M. Robert Knapp of the Minor Surgery Center of Wichita feels that controlling health costs is essential to preserving the free enterprise aspect of private practice. He and his colleagues have worked very hard to develop their freestanding independently operated ambulatory surgical facility.[1]

One investigator, Anne Somers, strongly recommends that hospitals should become the "hub" of health care delivery in the community.[2] Dr. Knapp argues that "that is not where it belongs. The result of that would be the reduction of the medical profession to a trade. . . ." He wants ". . . health care control out of the hands of hospital administrators and back in the hands of physicians." He further believes that "too few doctors are aware of the hospital's play for power and that it represents a distinct threat to the free practice of medicine."[3]

However, if doctors and hospitals fight it out, both will lose because the federal government is mapping out control plans right now, and it would behoove them to confederate and provide input into the system of controls facing them.

What about the alleged problem of hospitals charging too much for short-stay procedures? First, it should be noted that hospitals can lower charges because ambulatory surgery takes less time and facilities in the operating room. The "often charged" $200 for one hour of general surgery can be reduced to $100 for a typical short procedure. The one-day room rate can be eliminated since the patient doesn't use an inpatient bed—only a cot, and for only a very short time. The cost issue was developed in Chapter 4.

THE IMPACT OF SHORT-STAY SURGERY

As previously noted, many hospitals have viewed the advent of come-and-go surgery as competition to their surgery programs. Certain hospitals have modified their ambulatory surgical programs to take advantage of the market that independently operated programs have begun to capture.

In most cases, the surgical patients that an independently operated come-and-go surgical facility obtains are those involving private out-patient programs. To some extent, these are profitable surgical procedures because they are relatively minor in nature, requiring little in the way of sophisticated equipment and personnel to conduct the operation. In these cases, the ratio of revenue to expense is quite high.

Independently operated surgical facilities accept those patients that provide good medical risks, as well as good financial risks. This does not mean that excellent come-and-go facilities do not take on charity cases. They certainly do— especially the Surgicenter® in Phoenix. But, by and large, throughout the U.S., the high medical risk patients are left to be cared for by the hospital.

A Competitive Edge

It is important to note that ambulatory surgical centers tend to be anesthesiology centers rather than surgical centers because the key to an ambulatory surgery facility is the manner in which the anesthesiologists are available. When anesthesia coverage is available six days a week throughout the operating day, this creates many advantages for a busy surgeon who cannot always obtain such coverage at his local hospital. In the hospital setting, the surgeon has not only to coordinate the availability of the hospital bed and the operating suite, but also the limited time of the anesthesiologist. Many independently operated ambulatory surgery facilities allow for immediate patient access, waiting rooms for patients' relatives, and a pleasant relaxing atmosphere for patients, relatives and physicians. To the extent that this is not always available in the conventional hospital setting, we can say that competition certainly does exist.

The only time that competition doesn't exist is when the surgical facilities of the local hospital are taxed to capacity. This is often the case in some urban centers, but the question remaining is whether or not this will exist in the future. Will PSROs empty our nation's beds?

It is important for an independently operated program, as well as the hospital program, to have patient flow that is convenient and efficient from registration to preop, to surgery and recovery. The surgeon must be allowed to schedule in rather large blocks of time so that he can take maximum advantage of his own available time, and schedule one case to follow another. The need for travel time from one hospital to another is eliminated if he can perform in a well-organized independently operated facility, or in one hospital.

Can hospitals meet this challenge? Some may not; but more and more, we see hospitals across the country rising to this challenge.

The surgeon who is attempting to do come-and-go surgery must have his administrative requirements adequately provided for, and he must be able to step immediately from the operating room, dictate the operating note, and move on to the next case. He also must assist in gathering whatever information is necessary for billing purposes. This makes his use of time efficient and convenient.

Sometimes independently operated surgical facilities start out by performing very minor surgery and then begin to take on more cases of an increasingly sophisticated nature. As surgeons and anesthesiologists become increasingly familiar with this type of environment, they become more aggressive in terms of the level of surgery that they are willing to undertake.

This is where one sees a continuation of inroads that are reducing the surgical load of the nonprofit hospital. Hospitals have not always been responsive to this trend and are still bound with many of the old policy standards that are set down by hospital medical staffs, requiring inpatient hospitalization of patients for virtually all surgical procedures. Many hospitals in the U. S. today require that a patient coming into the hospital for a surgical procedure be admitted. If independently operated surgical facilities will perform those same procedures on an outpatient basis, we can readily see how competition will increase.

The independently operated surgical facilities are beginning to perform pediatric, plastic, GYN, and minor surgical procedures, all of which were previously done in a hospital setting. (See Appendix E.) Loss of these procedures can have a significant impact on the pediatric, OB-GYN and surgical programs of hospitals. Some hospitals have claimed that the impact of surgery being taken out of the hospitals tends to reduce the effectiveness of general medical-surgical programs within their organization.

Many offices constructed for physicians now contain outpatient surgical suites, and this trend is increasing. It is alleged that surgeons and anesthesiologists are acutely aware of the possible lucrative practice that outpatient surgery can provide.

Some hospital administrators have suggested that residency programs can be adversely affected by the decline of such surgery at their hospitals. Certainly, teaching programs want to see the major cases, but it is also important that they have the quantity of cases as well as the complexity needed to learn their skills.

The concept of come-and-go surgery places many challenges upon health care leaders to maximize community utilization of such surgery. Tradition-minded hospitals transfer short-stay surgical patients to a "recovery room." Since you "recover" from "sickness," and the independently operated facilities don't regard ambulatory surgery patients as "sick," they transfer patients to a "wake-up area." This is one of many of the creative innovations of the Minor Surgery Center of Wichita.

Hospitals are now receiving and will continue to receive many fiscal challenges as a result of new competition from nonhospital surgery centers. (See Appendix G.) How well will we administrators respond? My recommendation is that we concentrate on providing proper service to the community we serve and recognize that, under certain conditions, both approaches can coexist. This would leave us with only the cost issue to be researched and settled once and for all.

Notes

1. J. Floerchinger, "A Fight for the Right to Compete," *Private Practice*, August 1973; and M.R. Knapp et al., "Minor Surgery Center: An Answer to Escalating Costs," *Journal of the Kansas Medical Society*, December 1973, pp. 446-449.

2. Anne R. Somers, "Only the Hospital Can Do It All Now, "*Modern Hospital*, July 1972, pp. 95-102.

3. J. Floerchinger, op. cit.

Part IV
The Broad Issues in Ambulatory Surgery

The broad issues in ambulatory surgery are well developed in Part IV. The major viewpoints of the federal government are presented in the first chapter by Michael J. Goran, M.D., director, Bureau of Quality Assurance, Department of Health, Education, and Welfare, Washington, D.C., and Magruder C. Donaldson, M.D., of the Bureau of Quality Assurance. The emphasis here is on the role of quality assurance in health care delivery, with specific reference to ambulatory surgery.

John D. Porterfield, M.D., director of the Joint Commission on Accreditation of Hospitals, is the author of the chapter entitled "Joint Commission on Accreditation of Hospitals Accreditation Program for Ambulatory Health Care." He describes the overall issues in patient care and the role of the JCAH in insuring quality delivery of health care.

The Joint Commission has certainly been a bulwark of strength these many years through their educational efforts and their surveys of hospitals in maintaining the sound level of quality care that we now have in our American hospital system.

Some of the major cost implications are presented by Allen Weltmann, partner, Coopers & Lybrand in New York City, in his chapter entitled "Cost Determinations and Constraints in Ambulatory Surgery." He reveals the impact of Medicare regulations and the implication of embarking on ambitious programs of ambulatory surgery when inpatient occupancies are low.

Chapter 19 was prepared by the President of Blue Cross and Blue Shield of Michigan, Mr. John C. McCabe. In it he discusses the framework of the general problem facing American health care today: that the cost of care is reaching beyond the limits of acceptability. Third party payers, the federal government, and state governments are all amassing forces in an attempt to contain the rising costs of health care delivery. Mr. McCabe effectively examines these issues from a national standpoint. He points out that ambulatory surgery is a sound way to contain the mushrooming costs of health care delivery.

A major section of Part IV is reprinted from the Introduction to the Ambulatory Surgery Criteria and Standards Monograph prepared by Marie Erbstoeszer, University of Washington, for The Health Resources Administration, Department of Health, Education, & Welfare, Contract No.: HRA 106-74-56. This overall project is going to be published under the auspices of the U.S. federal government, and will serve a significant role in the evaluation of proposed ambulatory surgical programs by health service agencies throughout the U.S. The introduction describes the framework for the project and outlines some of the most important issues affecting ambulatory surgery in the U.S. today.

Bradley W. Yost, director, Health Care Policy, Blue Cross Association in Chicago, Illinois, wrote a chapter, "Blue Cross Association Perspective on Ambulatory Surgery." It presents a brief update of the philosophy of the national Blue Cross organization in regard to the delivery of care pertinent to ambulatory surgery.

The concluding chapter attempts to summarize the major conclusions of the entire book. It is our hope that no major areas affecting the delivery of care in ambulatory surgery have been overlooked. Every attempt was made to make this as complete as possible. While certain issues can be examined in more depth, our objective is to provide a well-rounded treatment of this important subject.

Chapter 17
Role of the Federal Government in Ambulatory Surgery:
Implications of Quality Assurance*

Michael J. Goran, MD and Magruder C. Donaldson, MD

Numerous reports in the literature indicate both enthusiasm and continuing debate on the impact of ambulatory surgery on society. It seems clear that the concept of "in-and-out," same-day surgery, as developed in its multiple forms across the country, represents a major potential for innovation in American health care delivery.[1-5]

From a societal point of view, perhaps the greatest impetus behind the ambulatory surgery concept is its potential for reducing the costs of services. This potential applies to both freestanding and hospital-based facilities, the two major prototypes for ambulatory surgery. By eliminating overnight hospital stays, expenditures for hospital services for inpatient health care, which now account for about 40% of our total national health expenditure, may be reduced directly and dramatically, at least on a short-term basis. By focusing on reducing inpatient surgery (accounting for 60% of all hospital expenditures and about 25% of total health care expenditures), ambulatory surgery may further reduce costs. By increasing efficiency and convenience, the surgeon may save time and, thus, be able to charge less for his services. Finally, with early and efficient treatment, patients may return to productive pursuits sooner, alleviating losses to the general economy.

Although direct savings to the patient and third party insurers can be documented as high as 60% according to one report, the long term economic impact of ambulatory surgery on the community is far from clear.[6] If a substantial proportion of the surgical procedures which are now performed in hospitals on an inpatient basis can be carried out effectively and safely in either freestanding or hospital-based ambulatory facilities, we must anticipate a substantial impact on the hospital economy. In communities where hospital inpatient facilities are

*Being published simultaneously in the August 1976 issue of *Hospital Progress,* published by The Catholic Hospital Association, St. Louis, Missouri.

overburdened with demand for surgical services, ambulatory facilities may provide valuable relief at a cost lower than would otherwise be incurred. However, in communities where the demand for surgical services is insufficient to fill all available hospital beds, addition of ambulatory facilities may exacerbate the hospitals' financial problems. The community, in turn, may find itself facing higher hospital rates to maintain additional unused beds. Closing those additional beds, or converting them to meet other real community needs such as long-term care, are possible alternatives, but such solutions to over-bedding have up to now been achieved only with great difficulty.

A related cost issue which is yet unresolved is the question whether the availability of ambulatory surgery facilities will cause an increased demand for procedures. Relocating present inpatient case load to an outpatient setting is one matter, but the possibilities of stimulating a rise in demand must be carefully considered as public policy towards ambulatory surgery is established. Closely related to this issue is an examination of mechanisms to eliminate procedures from the ambulatory surgery setting which are unnecessary and which can be adequately carried out in a doctor's office or clinic.

Local health planning agencies, such as those created by the National Health Planning and Resources Development Act of 1974 (P.L. 93-641), must play an important role in articulating community needs and guiding efforts to meet those needs. Their role is to balance the impact of ambulatory surgical facilities, whether freestanding or hospital-based, on the local economy against the demands and priorities of each community. The role of government, at least in part, is to assure that sufficient information exists to allow for informed debate and decision at all levels of public policy making.

Another major impetus for the development of ambulatory surgery has been its potential for improving quality of surgical care. Though cost issues are by no means clearly resolved, they may be more easily analyzed than the related issues of quality. We must be assured that creation of a new mode of surgical care delivery will—at the very least—maintain quality at the same level as the inpatient setting. Any improvements in quality related to ambulatory surgery must be carefully compared to possible detriments before we can unequivocally state that ambulatory surgery is *as* safe and effective as, let alone *more* safe and effective than, inpatient surgery. While concerned with expanding health expenditures, the federal government is equally concerned with the excellence of the health services the expenditures purchase. The prime goal of the government, and of society as a whole, should be to assure quality and to control waste, not cost, so that each service fully justifies its cost.

Supporters of the ambulatory surgery concept in its multiple forms have pointed out that large numbers of procedures can be performed under general anesthesia on a same-day basis with no detriment to the patient. Tonsillectomies, D&Cs and herniorrhaphies are among the various types of procedures which have been performed in ambulatory surgical units with complication rates that compare favorably with those for similar inpatients. In addition, patient acceptance of ambulatory treatment is high according to many published ·reports. Given adequate objective evidence of quality, patient opinion becomes an important quality consideration.[6-11] It is less clear whether ambulatory surgical facilities either increase or decrease the incidence of "unnecessary" surgery. While definitions of necessity may often be at variance with one another, this question clearly deserves further attention as a quality issue, since the risks of anesthesia and surgery should never be incurred needlessly.

If it is assumed, from preliminary evidence, that it is possible to maintain, and perhaps even improve, the quality of surgical care by an ambulatory setting, the primary issues before us relate to implementation of appropriate mechanisms to assure quality on an ongoing basis. What standards should be set for ambulatory surgery? Who should set them? How should standards be applied? To whom should ambulatory surgical units be accountable? What measures are appropriate to assure that standards are met? Fundamentally, of course, each member of the medical profession must be responsible for setting and implementing his own standards. A physician's training and ongoing experience shape his medical judgment into a tool which, more than any external device, has the potential for assuring quality performance. However, as health care becomes increasingly complex, it becomes more and more difficult for a single physician to remain abreast of the knowledge he needs and to maintain control of each element of the services which his patient receives. Typically, in a modern hospital, a patient may require the services of several specialized physicians and numerous ancillary departments, including nursing, respiratory therapy, anesthesia, laboratory, pathology, pharmacy and blood bank. Thus, the nature of modern medicine has compelled the providers of medical care to develop sophisticated methods of quality assurance. At the institutional level, tissue committees, morbidity and mortality conferences, grand rounds and audit committees have served this purpose, utilizing the concept of peer review to analyze, usually retrospectively, the results of health care. In addition, within the health professions on a national and regional basis, various certification, accreditation and continuing education activities have sprung up, and many specialty organizations have gone as far as to specify written standards of care for their members.

Beyond the impetus from within the profession, groups outside medicine have added unprecedented compulsion to quality assurance efforts. Third party insurers have legitimate concerns that they are getting quality in return for their expenditures. As sponsors of health care paid with taxpayer money, state and federal governments, more than ever before, are demanding assurances of quality. The demand is for more than the tacit approval of a committee of a physician's peers. Quality assurance today implies objective proof, clearly documented and accountable in public, that health expenditures are being used to provide services with maximum efficiency and safety. State governments have established licensure agencies whose function is to certify health care facilities and to assure compliance with standards of performance. The federal government, likewise, has set conditions which facilities must satisfy on an ongoing basis in order to participate in federal health care programs. The Department of Health, Education, and Welfare has established the Bureau of Quality Assurance to oversee the quality of federal health programs such as Medicare and Medicaid. With National Health Insurance, the federal role will increase, and the bureau's responsibility will likewise grow. Clearly, the federal government must seek accountability of quality from ambulatory surgical facilities no less than from other medical care facilities. It must also participate in promoting sound quality assurance programs in ambulatory surgery. We would like to focus on the quality issues previously mentioned and outline some of the current options and possibilities for their resolution.

The issue of setting standards for ambulatory surgery relates directly to the definition of ambulatory surgery and the ambulatory surgery facility. Though there are a variety of prototypes now operational, some general statements can be made. Ambulatory surgery implies completion of a procedure on a same day basis, without anticipation of overnight stay in a health care facility. Ambulatory surgery is distinct from surgery performed in a doctor's office or the usual outpatient clinic. Such surgery implies the necessity, in most cases, and the capability, in all cases, for anesthesia (local, regional or general). Ambulatory surgery is applicable only to carefully selected patients who are otherwise healthy and in whom serious complications are highly unlikely. Finally, ambulatory surgery connotes a capability for preoperative and postoperative care to assure proper outcome of the procedures which are performed. Given these general guidelines, we can discuss standards which will promote maximum quality of care rendered in ambulatory facilities.

Standards can be derived which relate to the structure of ambulatory facilities, to the processes by which they function, and to the results they produce. Structural standards should relate to the basic physical characteristics of the facility, including the safety and soundness of the actual plant itself. Structural standards should also address the availability and adequacy of special equipment (defibrillators and anesthesia machines), special resources, such as the capability for obtaining and administering blood products and medications and for providing pathology services. In addition, structural standards should include the organization, administration and staffing of the facility with properly qualified personnel, and should provide the capability for rapid and appropriate specialty consultation when necessary.

Process standards should relate to the manner in which ambulatory facilities function. Of vital importance here are considerations which will assure proper patient selection. Disease category, presence of complicating diagnoses, overall general health, patient attitude and family and social support are all relevant factors to be considered. Particular emphasis should be placed on assuring the medical necessity of each procedure. Proper patient selection standards should guarantee that the ambulatory facility does not overextend itself by providing services to patients who would do better as inpatients, or by encouraging provision of services to patients who can be managed adequately in a doctor's office or outpatient clinic. Beyond patient selection, process standards should guide each step of the preoperative evaluation and preparation for anesthesia and surgery, the surgery itself, and the immediate and longterm postoperative phases of care. Procedures for timely intervention by facility staff or consulting staff, including procedures for transfer to a back-up facility, should be specified.

Finally, outcome standards should state the general criteria of success which the facility will strive to attain. Included here should be goals relating to correlation of pathology reports with preoperative diagnosis, morbidity and mortality rates and levels of patient and physician satisfaction with their experience in the ambulatory facility. Outcome performance, of course, is the ultimate measure of excellence, and where outcome does not meet standards, structure and process standards should be altered or more strictly enforced to effect improvement. Though, in general, these basic standards for structure, process and outcome should be fundamental to all ambulatory facilities, there may be a different emphasis between standards applied to hospital-based facilities as opposed to freestanding facilities. Well-established standards for hospitals have evolved over a period of years to reflect the wide range of services available to the community and to accommodate the hospitals' particular institutional needs. Hospital associations at the state and national levels have become influential advocates of hospital interests. Hospital-based ambulatory facilities can expect to be subject, in large measure, to standards based on the precedents set for other hospital services.

Freestanding ambulatory surgery facilities, on the other hand, represent a significant departure from past experience. As institutions similar to hospitals in many respects, standards may be somewhat similar to hospital standards. However, we must be careful to recognize the unique characteristics and capabilities of freestanding facilities and to provide enough tailoring of standards to allow full realization for their potential. (New interest groups, such as the Society for the Advancement of Freestanding Ambulatory Surgery, must be recognized as valuable participants in resolving the issue of setting standards.) Who should set standards for ambulatory surgery? Government must continue to reserve the right to set and maintain conformity with standard as a condition of payment for services. At the federal, state and local levels, governments have in the past applied certain standards through survey agencies and facility licensure and certification boards, with emphasis on structural guidelines for hospital facilities. To date, few state governments have developed standards and licenses for freestanding ambulatory facilities, though many states are making progress in this area. The federal government, through the Bureau of Quality Assurance, has formulated draft guidelines for general ambulatory health care centers which are now being field tested. Ambulatory surgical facility standards are under consideration, but have not yet been fully developed.

Professional groups, such as JCAH, have also traditionally contributed to the process of standard setting, appropriately emphasizing guidelines relating to process and outcome of services. The JCAH is currently engaged in developing quality guidelines for ambulatory care, including ambulatory surgery. Other professional groups, such as the American Hospital Association and the American Academy of Medical Administrators have contributed significantly in the area of ambulatory surgery, and various specialty groups, such as the American College of Obstetricians and Gynecologists and the American Society of Anesthesiologists have also drafted standards. Consumer groups, involved primarily through input into government standards, are now concerned mainly with outcome standards and patient rights.

Clearly, standards should be agreed upon by everyone involved in ambulatory surgery, including government, third party payers, professionals, administrators and consumers. Much work remains to be done, particularly in the area of standards for freestanding facilities, and cooperation among all interests is essential to avoid duplication, contradiction and bias in favor of one particular form of ambulatory surgery over another. While certain aspects, such as structural standards, may be emphasized by some interests, other aspects, such as process standards, may be best left to professionals. In this regard, PSROs may provide a useful forum for voicing the concerns of government, third parties, professionals and consumers. Furthermore, PSROs are regionally distributed and can adapt standards to fit local conditions without sacrificing objectivity. Monitoring by the Bureau of Quality Assurance and the National Professional Standards Review Council can assure the soundness of PSRO standards. There are 120 PSROs in existence. Although all are still in their infancy, their potential for contributing in this area is great.

How can standards be applied? Precedents in quality review include traditional tissue committees, morbidity and mortality conferences, utilization review committees and audit committees. In addition, the JCAH surveys institutions regularly for accreditation, and state and federal agencies review compliance with standards every year.

Hospital-based ambulatory surgery facilities can easily be included in the activities of present institutional quality assurance peer review committees. Some freestanding facilities have established audit and tissue committees, based on the hospital model of peer review. On the other hand, freestanding centers may be small and compact enough to provide close quality review without need for separate committees. Requirements for quality review must not be unnecessarily burdensome when less time-consuming and less expensive mechanisms can perform adequately. More information on appropriate methods for review in freestanding centers is needed.

In the area of quality review, PSROs, again, may provide a useful mechanism. Since the PSRO program was initiated by Congress in the 1972 Amendments to the Social Security Act, 63 organizations have been funded to perform review in short-stay general hospitals. An additional 57 organizations are now in the planning stages, and eventually there will be 203 PSROs nationwide. As currently envisioned, these organizations, which include membership of all physicians in each local area, will review each Medicare, Medicaid and Maternal and Child Health Patient during his hospital stay. Objective, written standards will be used to assure the necessity and appropriateness of care rendered, as well as the quality of services. Retrospective audits, called medical care evaluation studies, will be performed regularly on topics of concern in order to identify areas of care where deficiencies in quality need improvement. Extensive data on each patient will be collected and carefully analyzed to indicate patterns of care for particular diagnoses, patterns of practice for particular physicians, and patterns of utilization for particular facilities. Though subject to strict rules of confidentiality, this data will be of extensive value to PSROs and their physician members in improving quality of care, and can also be made available to regional health planning agencies to assist in allocating resources for health care. As PSROs assume authority for hospital review, ambulatory surgery performed in hospitals can easily be incorporated into the PSRO system. Freestanding surgical facilities could, in principle, likewise participate in PSRO functions. At present, review of ambulatory services by PSROs is not required by law, but has been left optional, according to the desire of each PSRO. In addition, the PSRO mandate extends only to federal patients, though many PSROs are prepared to offer services to privately insured consumers. With time, and as National Health Insurance becomes a reality, PSROs will undoubtedly become a major instrument for applying standards of quality to freestanding, as well as hospital-affiliated, surgical facilities.

To whom should ambulatory surgical units be accountable and what measures are appropriate to assure that standards are met? Traditionally, individual physicans are accountable to themselves, to their peers and to the hospital board. Enforcement measures have included peer pressure for further education and changes in practice patterns as well as the extreme measures of removal from the hospital staff or delicensure. Institutions remain accountable to state and federal agencies and to the JCAH, subject to reduction or cessation of benefits under government programs. Ambulatory surgical facilities, whether hospital-based or freestanding, must remain accountable to external agencies and subject to appropriate improvement provisions and sanctions when deficiencies in meeting standards are identified.

PSROs, in addition to providing local physicians with a forum for setting standards and a tool for applying the standards and documenting performance, can focus continuing education efforts in the areas where problems exist. Being regionally-based rather than institutionally-based, PSROs can remain relatively objective in their activities, and public credibility should be high. Being professional organizations, the subtleties of medical practice can be adequately reflected in their judgments. At the same time they can avoid arbitrary and potentially dangerous consequences for facilities, physicians and patients. The result may be a beneficial decrease in the incidence of malpractice litigation.

The greatest need at this point is further articulation of standards for ambulatory surgery. Whereas hospital-based facilities may easily fit into the context of existing hospital standards, clear standards for freestanding centers are missing. Before this work is completed, issues of definition must be resolved. More information is necessary on the impact of ambulatory surgery on hospital patient load, the demand for services, the economy of hospitals and the community and on the quality of care. In the meantime, healthy competition and inquiry may stimulate improvement in services which are now widely available.

The federal government is highly interested in the potential of ambulatory surgery, and will continue to cooperate with efforts to resolve relevant issues. In addition to the potential impact of ambulatory surgery on federal health programs, the PSRO program and the new health planning legislation will become directly involved sooner or later.

Notes

1. Perspective 9 (3), 1974, pp. 1-17.
2. T.R. O'Donovan, *Hospital Administration*, Vol. 20, Winter 1975, pp. 27-39.
3. B.S. Epstein et al., *Hospitals*, Vol. 47, September 1973, pp. 80-84.
4. J. Calnan and P. Martin, *British Medical Journal*, October 9, 1971, pp. 92-96.
5. T.H. Berrill, *British Medical Journal*, November 11, 1972, pp. 348-349.
6. W.W. Funderbunk, *Journal of the National Medical Association*, Vol. 66, September 1974, pp. 416-419.
7. C.P.Shah et al., *Medical Care*, Vol. 10, September October 1972, pp. 437-450.

8. O. Echeverri et al., *International Journal of Health Services,* Vol. 2, 1972, pp. 101-110.

9. C.V. Ruckley et al., *Lancet,* November 24, 1973, pp. 1193-1196.

10. T.M. Chiang et al., *Archives of Otolaryngology,* Vol. 88, September 1968, pp. 307-310.

11. M. Levy and C.S. Coakley, *Southern Medical Journal,* Vol. 61, September 1968, pp. 995-998.

Chapter 18
Joint Commission on Accreditation of Hospitals
Accreditation Program for Ambulatory Health Care

John D. Porterfield, MD

More than 60 years ago the modern history of the assessment of quality of patient care began with the work of Emory Avery Codman, a Boston surgeon, and his associates. They were prime movers in the creation of the American College of Surgeons (ACS), and their interest in the analysis of patient outcomes led to the establishment in 1918 of the ACS's Hospital Standardization Program.

That program of standards development, hospital visitation and evaluation, and recognition of compliance with standards by accreditation is the basic pattern still supported by the Joint Commission on Accreditation of Hospitals (JCAH) since its founding in 1951. In that year the Commission assumed from the ACS the role of the health professions' voluntary "conscience" and self-improvement stimulator. The Commission was born as an independent, not-for-profit corporation sponsored by the American College of Physicians, the American Hospital Association, and the American Medical Association, in addition to the American College of Surgeons.

The basic philosophic concepts of Codman and his associates, which resulted in the founding of the ACS and its Hospital Standardization Program, may be stated briefly in three principles: (1) people should be qualified for the work they do; (2) the work environment and resources should be safe and functionally efficient; and (3) the quality of the work should be measured by its outcome. These concepts have been broadened and formalized in standards developed by the JCAH. The standards are constantly being reviewed and revised to reflect the state of the art of assessment of health care quality.

Since 1966, the JCAH has expanded the scope of its activities to offer standards and accreditation to other categories of health care and related services, in addition to the Hospital Accreditation Program. These categories now include long-term care facilities, facilities for the mentally retarded, psychiatric facilities, and, most recently, ambulatory health care. The accreditation process for all programs includes three basic elements: (1) the setting of optimal achievable standards of quality of care, (2) on-site surveys, including consulta-

153

tion; and (3) evaluation to determine (a) whether the facility is in substantial compliance with standards, (b) that there is no clear and immediate danger to patient safety and quality of care, and (c) that, in the case of a facility seeking reaccreditation, there has been progress toward better compliance with standards since the previous survey.

Until the late 1960s, the Hospital Accreditation Program concentrated on environmental and organizational aspects of institutions. Only more recently, as methodologies for measuring outcomes have been developed, has the profession—not to mention the patient and the provider—turned its attention to the quality of health care delivered. Thus, in April 1974, the JCAH Board of Commissioners approved a new section of the *Accreditation Manual for Hospitals* on the quality of professional services. In December 1975, the Board approved three new sections of standards replacing the previous single section on environmental services. The new sections include building and grounds safety, functional safety and sanitation, and infection control. This continuing process of development and revision of standards reflects the Commission's dedication to maintaining a leadership role in setting the health professions' goal as the optimal achievable quality of patient care.

Turning to the specific topic of the development of the Accreditation Council for Ambulatory Health Care, the JCAH has been actively engaged in consideration of such a program since 1970. The American Association of Medical Clinics (now the American Group Practice Association, AGPA) initiated discussions with JCAH to explore the feasibility of associating their accreditation program with programs of the Joint Commission. The AGPA Program was limited to formally organized group practices. During the ensuing months and years, the Commission met with most of the national organizations involved in some aspect of ambulatory care, and acted as a catalyst, giving support for the development of an appropriate accreditation council. In early 1974, a meeting of the AGPA, the American Hospital Association, the American Medical Association, the Group Health Association of America, and the Medical Group Management Association was convened for the purpose of exploring the development of a council. Subsequently, the JCAH Board of Commissioners approved naming the five organizations as charter members of the Accreditation Council for Ambulatory Health Care.

The developmental stages of the council are being supported in part by a $496,955 grant from the W. K. Kellogg Foundation of Battle Creek, Michigan. The three-year grant extends to April 30, 1978, by which time the council expects to be self-supporting.

The new council will recommend to the JCAH Board of Commissioners standards for the optimal quality of ambulatory health care, and will conduct on-site surveys to measure compliance with the standards by those programs that voluntarily seek accreditation.

As defined in the council's proposed bylaws, ambulatory health care is "health care delivered by or under the direction of licensed doctors of medicine and/or doctors of osteopathy to recipients who are not institutionalized for a period exceeding 24 hours." This could include freestanding clinics, ambulatory surgical facilities, and other special service institutions. At the present time, the council does not contemplate the accreditation of individual office medical practices.

At its founding meeting, the council requested that the AGPA continue its accreditation program until the council's program became operational. The council will use AGPA's standards and survey procedures as guidelines in the preparation of its own standards and procedures. It will attempt to have an operational program during 1976.

The AGPA Program was begun in 1968, and accredits some 150 formally organized group practices of three or more physicians. However, it is limited by design to one portion of the ambulatory health care field.

The decision of the AGPA to become a charter member of the JCAH's more broadly based Accreditation Council provides an opportunity for the council to benefit from the experience of an ongoing program.

The standards and procedures developed by the new council will be in accord with the same basic elements of all JCAH accreditation programs. The goal is that through accreditation, professionals may demonstrate their responsibility for and accountability to patients for the quality of care.

Chapter 19
Cost Determinations and Constraints in Ambulatory Surgery

Allen Weltmann

There is no question that the next decade will be the most challenging period that the hospital industry has ever faced. The establishment of the new Health System Agencies (HSAs) under the Health Planning and Resources Development Act of 1974, utilization review regulations, the advent of National Health Insurance and other regulating legislation, which will undoubtedly be signed into law by both federal and state governments, could create an atmosphere of survival of the fittest. Along with these problems, a new crisis has arisen which sooner or later will reach out and affect every provider of health services: the financial dilemma now facing local and state governments.

In order for these government entities to remain financially viable, their budgets will have to be pared down to equal anticipated revenues. One of the areas that will come under close examination is the welfare program. Several governmental agencies have already reviewed this area and have made decisions to eliminate selective services and freeze reimbursement for services at specified levels. This in itself will have a detrimental effect upon providers of health care services. But, as in the past, most institutions can survive this type of financial setback. However, what could be disastrous is the possibility of a cutback in welfare eligibility. If this happens, many patients who previously qualified for Medicaid assistance will no longer be eligible, and thus become a bad debt. Under our present reimbursement structure, these bad debts can only be recovered through self-paying patients, and there is a limit as to how high a given institution can raise its charges to cover this new cost. Consequently, institutions with marginal financial resources could be faced with bankruptcy. Inner-city hospitals could find themselves in the position of having 25% of their admissions become bad debts.

Institutions faced with this problem should begin to carefully re-examine their operations. Cost containment or reduction programs should be put into effect without delay. In many cases, institutions will be surprised to find that a "trimming of the fat" could lead to greater efficiency and improved patient care. The decisions that must be made by health care institutions will not be easy, but the problems must be faced and dealt with realistically.

What role do ambulatory short-stay surgical centers have to play in all of this? Actually, they could play a very important one. Most people interpret the phrase "cost containment or cost reduction programs" as the control or cutback of expenses or programs. However, successful business managers believe that cost reduction can be fully achieved through the creation of new programs which continue to offer the same services but at a lower cost. An ambulatory short-stay surgical center is such a program.

In establishing an ambulatory short-stay surgical center it is important to separate the measures of success between the medical and financial aspects. A short-stay surgical center can be medically successful if the program achieves all of its objectives, while at the same time it can be financially unsuccessful. Providers of health care services have normally one primary explicit objective and another implicit objective. The explicit objective is the delivery of quality health care to patients; the implicit objective is the ability to remain financially viable in order to continue rendering care to patients.

According to most of the literature on ambulatory short-stay surgical centers, if such centers are established in a given geographical area, overall health care costs could be reduced through the closing of unneeded hospitals, hospital wings and the reduction in the need for replacement beds. Although this may be theoretically true, in actuality it has been proven that it is very difficult, although not impossible, to get all the hospitals in a given area together to agree upon a mutual program. Consequently, most institutions make their own decisions regardless of the neighboring hospitals.

Institutions must carefully review the resulting financial implications of these short-stay centers. To begin with, it must be determined whether or not the patients that will be treated in this center are presently occupying a hospital bed. If the patient is, there must be careful consideration given to the financial effect of treating the patient as an outpatient rather than an inpatient. Some of the factors to examine are:

- What effect does an ambulatory short-stay surgical center have on census?
- If the census is expected to drop as a result of this program, what effect will a decline in census have on the per diem rate?
- Can the hospital sufficiently cover its fixed costs with a drop in census?
- Will the present operating room become underutilized as a result of this program?
- What effect does this program have on overall revenues and cash flow?
- How much of a capital expenditure must be made to establish this program and how will it be funded?

Another question that must also be resolved concerns third party reimbursement. Under the Medicare regulations, a short stay surgical program that does not keep a patient overnight will have its costs reimbursed under the outpatient formula. Accordingly, only 80% of the total costs attributable to the short stay surgical patients will be reimbursed. Under most short stay surgical programs, this will not be significant, since the majority of patients treated will be under 65 years of age and, therefore, not covered under Medicare.

Reimbursement for the care rendered to Blue Cross patients is more significant in that a relatively high percentage of patients treated will have Blue Cross coverage. Most Blue Cross plans have not yet established any firm policy with regard to reimbursement for short-stay surgical patients. Furthermore, many of the plans have demonstrated some degree of flexibility in this area and are willing to experiment. This being the case, any institution considering a short stay surgical program should contact Blue Cross while they are still in the planning stages.

In approaching Blue Cross, a hospital should be prepared to demonstrate the cost effectiveness of such a program. The documentation necessary to make a positive case involves:
- financial projections of the operating costs of the ambulatory surgical unit
- financial projections of the hospital's total costs before and after the opening of the ambulatory surgical unit
- comparisons of the costs per relevant surgical operation before and after the opening of the ambulatory surgical unit.

This information should be used to demonstrate to Blue Cross that the costs per operation for the relevant procedures are lower utilizing the in-and-out surgery concept. Furthermore, this documentation *should* support the argument that the hospital's total costs and cost per patient day will not be any higher than they were before establishing this ambulatory surgical unit. In other words, a hospital must satisfy Blue Cross that its costs will not be higher, but in fact, lower, and that the result will be a savings not only to the patient but to Blue Cross as well.

Once this premise has been established, a hospital should be in a position to negotiate a rate with those plans that do not already have a fixed policy with regard to reimbursement for short stay surgical patients. Obviously, the hospital should attempt to negotiate a rate based upon charges because, from a financial point of view, this is the most advantageous position. In lieu of this, the hospital, at a minimum, should settle for some rate above costs. Again, this is only possible once the hospital has demonstrated that the hospital's costs will be reduced as a result of the new unit.

A word of caution is necessary at this point. The Medicare regulations state that a provider cannot charge different prices for similar services. Most intermediaries have interpreted this to mean that a D&C performed in an ambulatory surgical unit must have the same price as a D&C performed in the operating suite. If this Medicare provision is strictly enforced, then a hospital would not be able to establish a lesser charge commensurate with the costs in the ambulatory unit. Accordingly, Blue Cross would probably not accrue any benefits if the operating room charge was established and paid by them for services provided through the ambulatory unit.

This problem, incidentally, of uniform charges for similar services not only affects short stay surgery but is creating a major obstacle in the treatment of all ambulatory patients. A hospital theoretically cannot charge a lower price to reflect lower costs for any ambulatory patient. Consequently, a contradiction exists between the regulations and the concern of government to reduce costs and charges.

If a hospital is planning to expand capital dollars in order to establish an ambulatory short stay surgical unit, it will be necessary to obtain Sec. 1122 approval and a certificate of need from the existing planning agency. Because health care planning is presently in a state of flux due to the new health planning law, there are no concrete criteria for determining the feasibility of establishing an ambulatory short-stay surgical center. However, a hospital should be prepared to supply the same information that was outlined earlier for Blue Cross purposes. Furthermore, there has been some evidence to date indicating that some planning agencies may require the hospital to give something up in return for approval of such a unit. In most cases, the agencies will look for a reduction in beds under the theory that an ambulatory short-stay surgical unit takes patients from an inpatient bed to an outpatient status, thereby leaving unfilled beds.

A counter-offer by a hospital could be to agree not to replace beds for a specified period of years and to review the need for a number of existing beds after that period. A hospital must be careful in negotiating a reduction in beds because, in all probability, once beds are taken away, it will be very difficult to get them back.

Too many institutions fail to include the hospital's top financial officer in the planning stages. His input before the fact could save the hospital money in structuring the unit through consideration of third party reimbursement rules. An example of a common mistake costly to many hospitals takes place in the building of a new structure for ambulatory services. If possible, it is more advantageous to remodel an older facility for ambulatory use and utilize a new structure for inpatient services. The reasons are that higher depreciation and interest costs will be allocated to the new inpatient facility, and, thus, third party reimbursement can be maximized.

In summary, ambulatory short-stay surgical units have a big place in our future health care system. But caution must be exercised in planning to protect the financial viability of the institution.

Chapter 20
Major Issues in the Total Escalation of Health Care Costs

John C. McCabe

The objective of this chapter is to explore ambulatory surgery as a major response to the problem of health care cost escalation. Because rising costs are a universal problem, they concern individuals, companies, and entire industries.

As president of one of the largest prepayment plans in the country (membership is 5.3 million persons), I am keenly aware that, while costs have risen generally, the health care industry has been the most heavily affected.

Consider the fact that in October the hospital care component of the Consumer Price Index was up 13.5% from a year earlier, compared with 11% for health costs generally, and just 7.6% for the CPI as a whole. In fiscal 1975, the nation's health bill reached $118.5 billion, a 13.9% increase in spending from fiscal 1974. This acceleration in health spending means that health care now accounts for 8.3% of the Gross National Product. Just 10 years ago it was 5.9%. This disproportionate increase over other spending is not just a phenomenon of the last year; it has been going on for at least 10 years.

How did the industry get into its present bind? First, our population has grown by 14 1/2 million from 1965 to 1972. The rising expectations of people apply to all areas of living, extending even to health care. How many times in the last few years have you heard the expression, "the right to health care?" It was not too many years ago that health care was considered a privilege, or at least a service for which the individual shared responsibility.

Inflation, which has hit all segments of the economy, is a large factor, especially in hospitals because they are labor-intensive. What does a $600,000 piece of equipment do to the operating costs of a hospital? That is the cost of a brain scanner, which is only a small part of the highly sophisticated technology that has developed in the diagnosis and treatment of illness.

Hospitals have larger staffs. In the seven year period from 1966 through 1972, the number of hospital personnel per 100 patients rose 60%.

The sharp escalation of professional liability premiums has played its role. Caspar Weinberger, former Secretary of Health, Education and Welfare, estimated that, in addition, the defensive practice of medicine, resulting from the threat of suits, has added from $3 to $6 billion yearly to the health bill.

There are obviously many facets to explain why health care costs have risen so sharply. The problem is complex and certainly the most pressing one that faces our industry today.

Last year our plan paid out $1.2 billion for health care services. Our payout as of September is running 17 1/2% ahead of the same period last year (with a slight reduction in enrollment). But we are not the only ones concerned. The concern is expressed in a variety of ways. In each of the last three sessions of Congress, bills calling for National Health Insurance have been introduced, a sure sign that some feel only government can put a brake on health care spending (although we know that government's entry into the health field through Medicare and Medicaid was one of the factors that fueled the flames of inflation in health care).

A poll published in October by the Cambridge Survey indicates that 57% of Americans support either a system of National Health Insurance or all-out socialized medicine. Only 13% wanted to preserve the status quo.

Business, big and small, is also concerned. A few months back, our largest customer, General Motors, called a special, unprecedented meeting of all its executives who hold public service jobs on hospital boards, Blue Cross and Blue Shield boards, and health planning groups to talk about what they could do to control health care costs. In addition, the auto companies and the United Auto Workers have agreed to set up separate company-union committees to search for ways of cutting these costs.

A recent meeting was held in Michigan of a joint legislative-governor's task force that is studying a redrafting of Michigan's health laws. It agreed in principle to ask the state legislature to create an independent Commission on Health Reimbursement, which would: (1) study how all health care agencies are paid for their services, including hospitals, nursing homes, and institutionally-based doctors; (2) conduct experiments in reimbursement to see if less expensive ways can be found to deliver needed health care in a variety of institutionally-related settings; and (3) draft and recommend legislation regulating payments and reimbursement policies of both state agencies and insurance companies.

Rate review legislation has already been enacted in eleven states and is pending in nine others. Although this legislation may raise cost awareness on the part of providers, there is not yet conclusive evidence that rate review is an effective hospital cost containment mechanism. This type of activity gives impetus to the cost containment programs already underway and to other programs being considered at Blue Cross and Blue Shield of Michigan.

I think our plan is fairly typical of the monetary stresses that have affected Blue Cross and Blue Shield Plans all over the country. Our membership has risen 7 1/2% from 1970 to 1974. This is equivalent to an additional 368,000 members for whom we are paying benefits. Because of increases in utilization of professional services and increasing costs per day for institutional care, our benefit payments during that period increased 51%.

Since the beginning of the year, we have been dipping into reserves at the rate of between $12 and $14 million per month. At this rate, we will reach a deficit by June 1976. To forestall this possibility, we have taken some extraordinary steps. These include a 10% cap over the 1975 level on all inpatient hospital reimbursement beginning January 1976 and continuing for a year. The cost cap will be retrospectively applied to total allowable inpatient costs before apportionment. In addition, those doctors who have had no profile increases granted since April 30, 1974, when federal controls were lifted, are eligible to apply for an increase of not more than 4%. The 4% is, in essence, a 10% cap since 40% of a physician's income goes for overhead expenses.

We will also be adopting other administrative changes: elimination of the professional handling charge for checking blood specimens; more stringent medical criteria for approving claims payments; and a more restrictive processing review technique to determine the medical necessity of diagnostic services.

Altogether, we hope to realize savings of $81.5 million. However, that will not alleviate our problem, so we have also filed for a 30.7% rate increase effective April 1976. I might point out that this is the result of inadequate rates approved by the state insurance commissioner for the past three years. For example, our rate increase request for the current year was cut in half. Moreover, the insurance commissioner figured into our rate allowance a 10% inflation factor for hospitals, when, in fact, this factor is running at about 20%. These latest programs add to the long-standing cost containment efforts which last year enabled us to reduce potential payout by $175.4 million, more than 15% of the total benefits paid out during the year.

Our regular and ongoing medical care cost containment programs fall into two areas: (1) physician reimbursement; and (2) the checks built into the claims processing system. We deal with more than 13,000 physicians. They are paid under the Michigan Variable Fee (MVF) contract, which reimburses physicians according to a "usual, customary and reasonable" formula. We maintain a profile of each physician's customary charges. Current charges are also tested against the prevailing screen, which represents the 90th percentile of charges by physicians of similar background and training. Prepayment screening of medical claims uses the computer to examine claims before payments to determine whether or not services rendered are covered by the contract; if the patient is a member under the contract; if the condition is pre-existing; if the charge exceeds any benefit maximum; if the kind and number of services are appropriate to the diagnosis; if there is a duplicate claim; if the same service for the patient was paid to another provider; and if similar services were rendered on the same date by other providers.

On the institutional side, an important effort had been the Hospital Qualifications Program. This establishes standards, places limitations on construction of new or expanded facilities including requirements for Certificate-of-Need under federal law, and requires accreditation by the JCAH and conformity with comprehensive health planning guidelines. We have also required that all participating hospitals conform with the decisions of comprehensive health planning agencies.

The leverage we had in these areas has been taken away from us through Certificate-of-Need legislation passed in the state, and accompanying legislation which stipulated that the corporation shall not deny participation on the basis of lack of community need.

Our reimbursement policy for participating hospitals assures that total costs are apportioned to accurately reflect the share of our members' care as a percent of total hospital costs. We conduct audits to be sure that only costs related to patient care are reimbursed, and that the lower rate of costs or charges is reimbursed. We use a mechanism designed to identify facilities with unusually high costs or large annual cost increases and to limit reimbursement which would otherwise be based on full cost.

Participating hospitals are grouped geographically and by size. Costs and percentages of cost increase throughout an institution's peer group are then calculated and compared, and those institutions which exceed the average increases receive limited reimbursement.

We try to control resource use through utilization review. Our representatives perform on-site compliance surveys for both Medicare and regular business cases. Particular attention is paid to the medical necessity of admissions, the appropriateness of services provided, the length of stay by diagnosis, under-and overutilization, and medical care evaluation reports conducted by the medical committees. Liability review, which assigns responsibility for payment where more than one carrier is involved, also saves money.

Overbedding is a serious problem both nationwide and locally. The Inter Study Group from Minneapolis issued a report indicating that with an 81% occupancy rate (using 1972 data) there are 60,000 excess community hospital beds nationally. Using that same occupancy rate and 1973 data, Michigan has about 1,207 excess beds. We are involved in a project to identify clearly overbedded hospital service areas in Michigan, and to develop appropriate corrective actions to bring bed supply more closely in line with need. The approach is on a case-by-case basis and provides for multilateral involvement of concerned parties. The success of the project will be evaluated in terms of the number of beds deactivated to provide a balanced supply that does not impair accessibility or curtail essential services. The latter considerations are extremely important. When government becomes involved in the problem, its approach is arbitrary and unilateral.

There are many other cost containment activities we undertake on an experimental basis. One is a tripartite pilot program agreed to by the auto companies, the United Auto Workers and our plan, for consultation on elective surgery. The program will provide additional surgical consultation by a qualified specialist(s) meeting program criteria for selected members who have been advised to have elective surgery.

Results of the program will be evaluated to determine its effect, if any, on surgical utilization and the health of the involved population, the cost effectiveness and cost containment potential, and the applicability of the program to the entire membership of our plan.

We are becoming concerned with the acquisition of expensive technical equipment that has not been fully tested and approved for particular application. Accordingly, in computerized transaxial tomography which performs brain and body scans, we will pay only for brain scans and then only when the scanner, either in or out of the hospital, has been approved by a planning agency. We will not pay for procedures of body scans until the clinical merits have been more clearly established.

Another way to contain costs is by covering alternatives to more costly inpatient care. This is a growing trend in Michigan and nationally. The Blue Cross Association reports that during fiscal 1974 ambulatory claims totaled 17.4 million, almost twice the 9.9 million claims for inpatient hospital admissions. The American Hospital Association notes that for fiscal year 1975 outpatient visits to community hospitals increased by 7.6% over the previous year. By contrast, admissions increased only 1.8%.

Michigan is no stranger to the concept of outpatient ambulatory surgery in the hospital environment. It was pioneered in Michigan at Butterworth Hospital in Grand Rapids in 1961. Since that time, the concept has flourished so that more than 2,600 of the 7,000 U.S. hospitals now offer one-day surgery.

Our plan has paid for all surgical care since its inception in the late 1930s. We have not, however, made any special additional payments for such surgical care in freestanding non-affiliated ambulatory facilities, and that may be one of the reasons that the growth of such facilities in Michigan has been limited.

Because we are always eager to explore any programs that may cut costs, we are currently talking to three groups of physicians who plan to operate, or are already operating freestanding ambulatory surgical facilities. Under three pilot projects, we will pay the additional facility costs of these groups.

Before entering into final agreement with the groups, we have laid down some stringent guidelines for them: the facility must be approved as to need by the appropriate planning agency; it must be licensed by the state of Michigan, accredited by the JCAH or the American Osteopathic Association; it must have a transfer agreement with a nearby hospital; and it must have appropriate professional review committees.

At the end of a period not to exceed two years, we hope, through these projects, to be able to evaluate costs, quality of care, utilization patterns, and the need for surgical facilities. We also hope to find answers to other questions: Might surgeons be tempted to perform procedures that should be done properly only in a hospital?; Would doctors switch the minor procedures they had done regularly in their offices to the more expensive freestanding facility?; Would the lack of certificate of need legislation in Michigan permit a proliferation of freestanding facilities in areas already overbedded?

Our plan this year will pay out an estimated $1.36 billion for some 30.8 million claims. We have a responsibility to our members to be sure that surgery outside the hospital is cost effective on an overall basis before we wholeheartedly endorse it.

I might add that there is a politically-motivated aspect to the question which has nothing to do with either costs or quality of care, i. e., the question of control of facilities. Should they be hospital-controlled? If not, how is high quality to be maintained? Part of the problem lies in the revenue-oriented position of the hospital administrator. By the same token, groups of physicians are often profit motivated and their goals may well be self-serving.

We at Blue Cross and Blue Shield of Michigan do not feel we have the final answers on cost containment, nor do we feel that we alone have responsibility for these endeavors.

Hospitals, because they represent the source of the greatest rise in health care costs, will have to be diligent in developing programs to contain or cut costs. For example, they can achieve better utilization of testing facilities through preadmission testing and by keeping x-ray and lab facilities open on weekends. They can do more to pool their facilities. Five northwest Detroit hospitals, formerly in competition with one another, have pooled their resources, offering the same services at reduced costs. Hospitals must continue to innovate, as in ambulatory day surgery.

As rooms, wards, and even entire floors are closed—as they surely must be—imaginative uses must be found for these resources. Many hospitals could embrace one-day surgery in their closed operating rooms. Doctors' offices can be moved into empty floors. On the other hand, there may well be times when the most efficient use of unnecessary space is to put excess facilities into moth balls against a future time when community needs may change.

Doctors must also put their efforts behind the reduction of health care costs. The community must pitch in to help solve malpractice problems, which result in defensive, and more expensive, medical care. Our plan is working with the Michigan Hospital Association and the state medical society for legislation that would improve the malpractice situation. Physicians must police their ranks to get rid of incompetent doctors who can cause professional liability suits. They must practice medicine as they know they should, making sure that each patient test, in and out of the hospital, is necessary. They must ensure that each surgical procedure is necessary, and determine whether earlier ambulation is possible in inpatient surgery.

There is still another area barely touched where savings could be realized—patient education. Pilot programs done with asthmatics, hemophiliacs, and diabetics show that educating these patients about their health problems can save $6 in health care for every $1 spent in education. A test program done with 97 patients facing abdominal surgery indicated that those educated about postoperative problems asked for fewer narcotics and were sent home an average of 2.7 days earlier than an uneducated group.

Much morbidity and mortality today results from our life styles. Somehow, we must get the message across that smoking, drinking, overeating, and lack of exercise have a bad effect on our health.

Similarly, much of our senior citizen's debility may stem from our current attitude that at the age of 65 we retire from life. Old people do become chronically ill, but putting them into nursing homes is not only expensive but tends to exacerbate their problems. A Blue Cross Association study noted that at least $200 million a year now being spent on nursing homes could be saved with viable home care programs, which incidentally do far more to preserve the dignity of senior citizens.

Unless some creative resolutions actually occur, there will be unilateral actions imposed on all segments of the industry by several entities, such as our plan and its Cost Reduction Program. We do, after all, present a mechanism by which public frustration is vented.

Whatever your professional affiliation, get involved. If your group doesn't have a cost containment committee, start one. Get together with other groups in your area and in other areas. In Michigan, the state medical society has designated a cost containment group that works closely with our plan. As individuals, we can do only a little to solve the problem of costs. Working in concert within our group, and joining with other groups, we can accomplish much more. Indeed, we must. It is quite simply a matter of survival. If we do not act as members of the private sector to control costs, the ability to act will not remain in our hands, but will go to government by default.

Chapter 21
The Health Services Criteria Project

Marie Erbstoeszer

This chapter provides an overview of the current issues frequently cited in regard to ambulatory surgery. Since clinical trials are difficult to conduct on human subjects, very few evaluations using sound experimental design have been reported.

The issues are grouped into the following categories: patient considerations; physician and surgeon considerations; implications for quality; impact on the utilization of health resources; and cost considerations. The purpose of the discussion is to give health systems agencies background information on the currently prevailing issues regarding ambulatory surgery.

PATIENT CONSIDERATIONS

Some patients find ambulatory surgery more acceptable than inpatient surgery.

Discussion: For surgical patients who do not require continuous professional postoperative observation and care extending beyond the same day of surgery, recovery in the home setting may be more convenient and agreeable. Often these patients resume their normal activities sooner and, therefore, the whole event may be less traumatic and life disruptive. This is particularly important for pediatric patients. The patient's personal feelings about ambulatory surgery must, however, be considered, since not all patients accept this concept. The adequacy of the home environment is also a critical factor in determining patient suitability for ambulatory sur-

*Reprinted from the Ambulatory Surgery Criteria and Standards Monograph prepared by Marie Erbstoeszer, University of Washington, for the Health Resources Administration, Department of Health, Education, and Welfare, Contract No.: HRA 106-74-56, 175.

Some patients are apprehensive about ambulatory surgery.

Discussion: Ambulatory surgery is not appropriate for all patients. It is a concept many patients are unfamiliar with and, therefore, may be apprehensive about. More specifically, patients may be reluctant to having surgery on an ambulatory basis for the following reasons:

(1) Not all patients, in spite of appropriate preoperative counseling, are good psychological candidates for ambulatory service.

(2) Often patients do not have anyone to take care of them at home and are frightened of the immediate discharge after surgery.

(3) Some patients live in areas without immediately accessible medical facilities. They fear discharge after surgery and the possibility of resultant complications with a lack of readily available medical resources.

(4) Patients fear that their insurance will not cover all costs such as the ancillary services or follow-up services.

(5) Patients feel that they are entitled to inpatient care.

PHYSICIAN AND SURGEON CONSIDERATIONS

Ambulatory surgery generally provides for the more efficient use of physicians' time, as compared with inpatient surgery.

Discussion: An efficiently organized ambulatory surgery unit has the potential of saving time and increasing convenience for physicians and surgeons by using a time-specific surgery schedule; by eliminating pre- and postoperative inhospital visits; and by reducing the amount of paperwork since less extensive records may be acceptable for ambulatory patients.

Physicians are often attracted to ambulatory surgery units or facilities because the professional staff is usually trained and skilled to meet the special needs of the physicians, the surgeons, and the ambulatory patients.

Discussion: Since these units or facilities provide services designed specifically for ambulatory surgery, the staff may be more adept, efficient and responsive to the particular needs of physicians, and ambulatory patients. The actual realization of this factor is dependent upon the characteristics of each individual ambulatory surgery unit or facility.

Some physicians are apprehensive about participating in the provision of ambulatory surgery services.

Discussion: Physicians may choose not to perform ambulatory surgery for several reasons:

(1) Fear of malpractice suits if they do not admit their patients to a hospital for surgical procedures. (With the current emphasis on malpractice insurance, this is a very important concern to physicians and surgeons. Very few lawsuits, however, have been reported to date in regard to complications following ambulatory surgery.)

(2) Fear of complications and lack of proper professional management after the patient is discharged and returns home.

(3) Concern about the lack of immediate hospital backup at freestanding facilities. (This concern can be alleviated if the facility has appropriate emergency capabilities.)

(4) Concern that the staff in the ambulatory surgery unit or facility is insufficiently skilled. (An example may be a unit or facility which does not see a high volume of ambulatory surgery patients and, therefore, cannot remain proficient in skills.)

(5) Concern that the staff in the ambulatory surgery unit or facility is over specialized in just one particular area of procedures, e.g., performing only gynecological procedures. Since physicians could not bring all of their ambulatory patients to this unit or facility, they may avoid it completely.

(6) Reluctance to bring patients to a physician-owned freestanding ambulatory surgery facility if they are not allowed to participate in the facility's profit sharing.

(7) Reluctance to bring patients to a surgeon-owned facility because they fear losing their patients to other surgeons.

IMPLICATIONS FOR QUALITY

Ambulatory surgery patients may experience less exposure to contamination and cross infection.

Discussion: While this opinion is frequently cited in the literature, it must be considered subjective, since no clinical trials have proven this hypothesis. The issue of exposure to contamination and subsequent infection depends upon a combination of factors: the relative aseptic control of the unit or facility; how well patients are isolated from potential sources of infection; and, of course, the patient's health status and potential immunity. The basic issue underlying this statement is how the service is provided, rather than whether or not the patient is ambulatory.

Ambulatory surgery patients may receive less medication—both pre- and postoperatively—than patients undergoing similar surgical procedures as inpatients within a hospital setting.

Discussion: The implications of this statement are frequently debated. While some professionals argue that less medication is better for patients, others maintain that patients receiving less medication may feel more discomfort after discharge. The actual relationship of the medication issue to quality is unresolved at present. The medication issue is basically related to two different systems of care. In the ambulatory setting a patient must be alert and prepared for discharge sooner than an inpatient. In an inpatient setting, the patient is under professional supervision for a longer period of time, and, thus, can receive more medication.

The safety of patients is assured when ambulatory surgery is performed in properly developed and controlled settings.

Discussion: Current experience and available data indicate that ambulatory surgery is a safe procedure when appropriate standards of care are enforced. Unfortunately, no uniformly accepted standards of quality control exist for ambulatory surgery services at the present time.

IMPACT ON THE UTILIZATION OF HEALTH SERVICES

Ambulatory surgery services allow the waiting time for elective surgery to be greatly reduced.

Discussion: The relevance of this statement is dependent upon whether there currently is a backlog of elective operations. The backlog may be a function of two factors, a limited hospital bed supply or a surgeon shortage. If there has been an extensive waiting period for hospital beds, ambulatory surgery may reduce the waiting time because: (1) some patients can then have their surgery performed on an ambulatory basis and avoid the wait or (2) the new ambulatory surgery service may reduce the demand for beds, and, thus, the waiting period for those patients who require hospitalization may be reduced. If the backlog is related to a surgeon shortage, ambulatory surgery may help by reducing the surgeon's time per procedure, thus allowing for the performance of more surgery.

Ambulatory surgery services free hospital beds and staff for more seriously ill patients.

Discussion: Like the preceding statement, this argument is dependent upon the current utilization and demand for hospital beds. The important overall issue, however, is the provision of the appropriate level of quality care for each patient's needs. The decision of whether to implement ambulatory surgery services should not be dependent on hospital bed utilization. If ambulatory surgery services cause an excess of unused beds, the proper solution should be to find alternate uses for the existing resources or to close the units and reallocate staff as necessary.

In those units or facilities organized strictly for ambulatory surgery, the patient receives more specialized and personal care.

Discussion: Since these units or facilities are providing service for only one type of patient, their operational efficiency may be greater than in settings where both inpatients and outpatients are seen. The personnel can focus their attention on one type of patient, and, therefore, provide care which is specific to the needs of the ambulatory patient. There may be a cost trade-off for this special care, however, if it results in underutilized and duplicate facilities.

Some facilities have positive attitudes toward ambulatory surgery but cannot implement such programs because their facilities and staff cannot be extended to meet the program requirements.

Discussion: Many people feel that any hospital with a surgical suite has capabilities of offering this service. There are, however, circumstances which make ambulatory surgery unfeasible for some hospitals:

(1) Space is lacking for patients' dressing facilities and bathrooms.
(2) Holding space for waiting preoperative patients is not available, and staff are not available to provide the required preoperative services.
(3) The operating room schedule is tight and cannot control delays or emergency-urgent scheduling requirements, making it impossible to guarantee ambulatory patients a specific surgical time.
(4) Recovery room facilities are inadequate to provide a non-threatening environment for patients.
(5) The hospital may be unable to have the statement of charges ready when the patient is discharged. Ambulatory surgery patients, once discharged, cannot be allowed to wait in the hospital. Many will have some degree of pain after arriving home, and surgeons wish to make sure that any such discomfort occurs only after the patient is in a safe environment.
(6) The hospital staff (including physicians and nurses) may be resistant to the development of ambulatory surgery.
(7) The area has too few patients who can be classified as probable ambulatory surgery candidates, thus prohibiting the development of a financially feasible service with adequate quality controls. If the demand for ambulatory surgery is too low, the unit or facility will not be able to hire or assign adequate staff for the appropriate management and operation of the service.

COST CONSIDERATIONS

Through the provision of ambulatory surgery services, the expense of two or three days of hospitalization can be averted.

Discussion: Generally, it is stated that ambulatory surgery patients are spared the expense of the room charge plus the routine inpatient charges which take place during the two to three days of hospitalization. However, the issue of actual community-wide cost savings has not yet been fully evaluated. A great deal of debate exists regarding this issue, and opinions vary widely.

A frequent point of confusion in the debate over economic implications of ambulatory surgery is the lack of distinction between costs and charges. Charges are the amount billed to the patient or the insurer. The cost is the actual amount which the provider must expend in order to supply the service. Although some providers may attempt to make charges as comparable to costs as possible, they have not often achieved this. When costs are compared, it must be made clear what is actually being compared (i.e., the actual costs, the exact same services). Since the cost/charge distinction often is not clarified, many of the existing reports are inconclusive.

Problems are also frequently encountered when trying to compare ambulatory surgery costs of hospitals with those of freestanding facilities. The charge for ambulatory surgery performed in a hospital may include a contribution to the hospital's relatively high overhead costs. The same surgery performed in a freestanding facility will not include these high overhead costs, and, therefore, should result in a lower charge to the individual patient. However, the cost of maintaining the hospital remains the same, and someone, other patients or the community, will have to pay such overhead costs unless the hospital closes. If no other inpatient facilities are available to the community, this can be a very serious consequence.

Ambulatory surgery patients generally receive screening exams which are appropriate for their specific type of surgery, thus avoiding the additional expense of tests routinely given to inpatients.

Discussion: When this policy is implemented, it results in a savings of dollars and of the patient's and the physician's time. The overall relevance of the statement, however, is dependent upon the standing orders which currently exist and the judgment of the physicians involved.

Ambulatory surgery may cause an increase in the charges or costs for inpatient surgery.

Discussion: As increasing numbers of patients are treated on an ambulatory basis, the case-mix of the hospital ward will change to include more serious surgery cases and more elderly patients, who require heavier medical and nursing care. Hospitals will then have cases which are on the average more costly. By itself this may not be a problem. Indeed, the change could result in more efficient utilization of hospital staff who are trained and paid to work with more difficult cases.

However, the shift could present a problem in those hospitals which have historically charged minor surgery cases above the actual cost in order to subsidize more complex surgery. Such hospitals will have to raise prices, and patients with complex problems, or their insurers, will have to pay more. The shift in case mix could also be a problem for a hospital if the same overhead costs have to be allocated to fewer cases. Individual hospital cases will have to pay a greater share of the overhead costs. One of the economic arguments in favor of independent ambulatory surgery units has been that they avoid overhead costs which are necessary only for medically complex cases.

Some third party payers do not fully reimburse for a surgical procedure which is done on an ambulatory basis.

Discussion: Generally, third party payers pay the physician charge for ambulatory surgery; the facility charge, however, may not be reimbursed if the patient is seen on a strictly ambulatory basis. These same third party payers will reimburse the complete (physician and facility) charge if the surgery is performed on an inpatient basis. When this situation prevails, there is an incentive to hospitalize patients. Some insurers do offer special "riders," at an increased premium, which include coverage of ambulatory surgery.

Some third party payers are reluctant to add ambulatory surgery as a benefit to their insurance policies because they do not know what the cost impact will be.

Discussion: Because the impact of ambulatory surgery on the total demand for health services is still unknown, third party payers are uncertain whether they should add the benefit without a premium change. Many insurers argue that any health resource which exists will be used and, therefore, the beds which are emptied by ambulatory surgery patients will be filled by other patients. If ambulatory surgery causes the demand for services to increase, it may result in premium increases. If, however, ambulatory surgery causes a decrease in the utilization of inpatient services, it may allow a decrease in premiums.

Ambulatory surgery relieves the demand for and pressure on inpatient facilities.

Discussion: Ambulatory surgery services should reduce the demand for inpatient beds. A savings in future capital expenditures for new health facilities may, therefore, be realized. Examples of these savings have been reported by the Comprehensive Health Planning Council of Maricopa County, Phoenix, Arizona, and the De Graff Memorial Hospital in North Tonawanda, New York.

The decreased demand for hospital beds may cause the closing down or alternate use of unneeded beds. Hospitals whose occupancy rates are below 80% are resistant to any plans for the provision of ambulatory surgery in their service areas. The ambulatory surgery procedures are seen as a threat to the hospitals' much-needed room revenues, which are bolstered by keeping the patient, at the very least, overnight. A number of important policy issues should be considered when this situation arises. First, planning for health services should have the goal of providing the appropriate level of care for each patient's needs. Keeping beds occupied by patients who do not require hospitalization is an inappropriate use of resources. There may, however, be some special contraindications to this approach in isolated areas. An example might be a small rural hospital which is the sole source of hospital services for a particular area. If the hospital already has a low or marginal occupancy rate, any further reduction brought about by ambulatory surgery may be the crushing blow which forces the closure of the hospital. Subsequently, the area might be completely without needed health services. The policy implications of the planning decisions must be carefully evaluated in each circumstance.

Chapter 22
Blue Cross Association
Perspective on Ambulatory Surgery

Bradley W. Yost

Because of the unique legal nature of Blue Cross Plans through their incorporation under special state statutes as nonprofit community service organizations, they have assumed certain responsibilities in the public interest. These responsibilities have been translated into a primary goal for the Blue Cross organization, which is to assure that our subscribers obtain sufficient amounts of acceptable quality health care at least possible cost. From this primary goal stem two basic operating objectives. The first is to assure the cost effective administration of health care insurance benefits to subscribers. Functions falling under this category include the normal insurance functions of marketing, accurate assessment of risk, claims payment, uniform interpretation of benefits, etc. In addition, another function receiving much greater attention these days is the provision of cost effective benefit offerings to our subscribers. Critics of the health care financing mechanism have argued that both government and private health insurance and prepayment programs have focused too much attention in the past on hospital acute care services, to the point where such coverage had (1) become a key factor contributing to the increased demand for, and cost of, hospital inpatient services, and (2) created a financial *disincentive* for the use of alternative medically appropriate yet lower cost services. Cost and utilization experience stemming from the Medicare program serves as one primary illustration to support this criticism. In response to this and other factors, the Blue Cross organization in recent years is increasingly reassessing its benefit programs, with the result that benefit coverage has been expanded to cover not only inpatient acute care services, but also services which can serve as lower cost alternatives to inpatient hospital care. Examples of such programs are: the provision of benefits for preadmission testing, outpatient diagnostic and therapy services and home health care.

The second basic operating objective for the Blue Cross organization is to help assure that the health care services received by Blue Cross subscribers are delivered in a medically appropriate and cost effective manner. Aside from,

179

but supportive of, what may be accomplished through innovation in benefit offerings to promote a more cost-effective health care delivery system, Blue Cross Plans throughout the country have actively developed and promoted various other innovative programs—in concert with providers—in the areas of utilization review, prospective reimbursement, HMOs, and health planning to help achieve the containment of health care costs and to assure that the services provided are medically appropriate and of acceptable quality. Within this context, ambulatory surgery, as a needed and desirable form of health care, is receiving greater recognition and insurance coverage by Blue Cross Plans throughout the country. In recognizing outpatient surgery as a desirable service for insurance coverage, Plans should address these two basic questions: (1) does ambulatory surgery generally fulfill the conditions of being cost-effective and providing quality care; and (2) if so, under what conditions or circumstances? In and of itself, experience to date would indicate that the concept of ambulatory surgery satisfies the requirements of technical quality. The American Medical Association, along with other professional associations, has endorsed the concept of ambulatory surgery under general and local anesthesia for selected procedures, on selected patients, as good medical practice. However, other aspects of quality medical care stretch beyond the issues of technology, including such factors as patient satisfaction, ease of access to care, continuity of care and comprehensiveness of care. The impact of ambulatory surgery on these parameters of quality are less certain, since they are largely dependent upon the locus of care: whether the surgery is performed within the hospital, adjacent to a hospital, in a hospital-affiliated satellite, or in a freestanding center.

As for cost considerations, it is obvious that a surgical procedure done on an outpatient basis which traditionally had been done on inpatients (requiring a one or two day length of stay) will cost the patient less in terms of total charges for the surgical procedure and related stay. However, as is true in many areas, cost analysis is not that simple. Again, the analysis must include several considerations, including the setting in which care is provided and the invested health care capital structure of the community. Thus, the concept of ambulatory surgery itself is not controversial, but the setting, hospital or freestanding, in which it is performed is.

There is little doubt that the widespread attention being given to ambulatory surgery, particularly when done in the freestanding setting, is largely due to the potential for reduction of health care costs. This cost reducing effect is often demonstrated by comparing total charges to the patient for various surgical procedures done in various settings. However, charge or cost comparisons of specific service units from one facility to another cannot fully substantiate cost savings effects. One reason is that prices often bear little discernible relationship to actual costs, particularly for hospitals. Also, a comparison of costs between two types of facilities must account for differences in range and intensity of services on both an inpatient and outpatient basis. This should include consideration for not only direct operating costs, but stand-by costs and the costs of a 24-hour operation. The best indicator is a close look at the total cost of a health care delivery system to the community. The transfer of medically appropriate services from an inpatient to an outpatient basis can serve to reduce community costs only if accompanied by commensurate adjustments in the existing capital structure and operating behavior of facilities. It must be recognized that inappropriate utilization of the existing facilities, any resulting idle capacity, or unnecessary facility additions, can nullify some or all of the cost savings potentially achieved through the increased use of ambulatory surgery. This fact must be taken into consideration not only in structuring the delivery system, but also in choosing the optimal locus for ambulatory surgery in any given community. Because of the many variables involved, the results of a cost analysis of this nature will most likely vary from one area to another, depending upon the individual circumstances involved.

The official position of the Blue Cross organization recognizes the need for increased coverage for certain types of ambulatory care, including ambulatory surgery. In addition, the Blue Cross organization has officially recognized the potential advantages and disadvantages of ambulatory surgery performed in various settings, and feels that the issues raised by the freestanding type facility must not be allowed to stand unresolved. The Association has encouraged Plans to proceed with formation of initial contractual relationships with freestanding ambulatory care facilities in the interest of supporting innovation accompanied by sound planning and evaluation. However, we also strongly believe that these relationships should fulfill certain conditions: the facilities should be part of an areawide health plan and be certified as to need or approved by the appropriate health planning authority; and the facilities should also meet various standards equivalent to those for hospitals in order to assure quality of care. This means complete, modern facilities and equipment, adequate numbers of skilled professional and technical personnel, maintaining detailed medical records and a strong working relationship with one or more hospitals to which patients needing additional care can be admitted promptly. There is a need for either states or the federal government or voluntary agencies to further pursue licensure and/or accreditation for freestanding centers in order to maintain the quality standards of care.

In summary, the concept of ambulatory surgery is receiving increasing recognition and financing from Blue Cross Plans. Although certain questions involving the advantages of ambulatory surgery have been sufficiently resolved, several questions need additional discussion and exploration. It is the job of both providers and insurers in the future to work cooperatively together to help resolve these issues and achieve an objective atmosphere of evaluation.

Chapter 23
Summary and Conclusion

Thomas R. O'Donovan

Now that the full gamut of ambulatory surgery has been brought forth, dissected, and completely analyzed, do we really have the final answers and know just what to do? At best, we have only a good start because more research is needed. Power-plays exist everywhere: hospitals doing ambulatory surgery versus the independents; federal government versus hospitals and physicians; consumer groups versus providers; one professional group versus another, etc.

In Chapter 4 we found many approaches to cost, but didn't learn how many specific dollars ambulatory surgery can save in the nation's health care bill. We discussed how ambulatory surgery will reduce "long-run" health care costs, yet in Chapter 17 ambulatory surgery is said to reduce health costs "at least on a short-term basis." Perhaps both statements are true depending on the definition of terms, but much clarification is needed.

We should examine carefully any sweeping statements and conclusions regarding any phase of health care delivery, including ambulatory surgery. One hears that 50% of all pediatric surgery can be performed on an ambulatory basis, but can this be documented? A federal government report recently said 25% of all surgery can be ambulatory, while others have claimed 50% or 40% or some other number. We must not assume facts without data.

Much value can be obtained from examining the chapters presented by the faculty of the American Academy of Medical Administrators (AAMA) conferences on Ambulatory Surgery as herein presented. The case studies will have special value because they give actual accounts of experiences of a range of hospitals with ambulatory surgery. Some of the hospitals have taken different approaches than others. Some of the material may appear to be duplicated. In many cases major concepts are similar, though different words are used to describe these concepts because the faculty of the AAMA conferences are from *all over* the U.S. and Canada. It is quite refreshing to note that there are very few inconsistencies. For the most part, there is definite agreement on the major concepts of ambulatory surgery. A few exceptions exist, which show that there is a role for research in the area of ambulatory surgery to resolve areas of disagreement.

We have mentioned several times the importance of research in ambulatory surgery. For example, in order to decide the impact on cost that would result from a hospital or independently operated facility embarking on a program of ambulatory surgery, consider the following situation: If a particular hospital in 1975 opened its ambulatory surgery unit and performed 1,000 procedures, we would have to know quite a bit of information before we could begin to determine what cost savings resulted. For example, how many of these 1,000 procedures would have been done in a hospital on an inpatient basis? How many would have been done by doctors in their offices, in an emergency room, in an outpatient clinic, or in another hospital facility or freestanding facility? How would you obtain that information? If you ask the doctors, they might be reluctant to reveal complete information because it might not be readily available, or for other personal reasons.

Nevertheless, the above information is important to obtain, otherwise you will not know whether you are reducing costs or shifting costs. It's the old problem of community costs versus costs incurred by an individual hospital. All of this information is difficult to obtain because the medical records department would not readily have such data for these cases. Some information can be obtained from the direct interview with patients, but even they might not know where their procedures would have been done if it hadn't been done in a hospital. Interviewing the doctor would be the most valid approach.

The AAMA pledges its continued cooperation in providing additional conferences and seminars on the subject of ambulatory surgery on an ongoing basis. Health care delivery in all its forms is going to receive many challenges in the years ahead. Perhaps, our greatest challenge will be how to deliver quality care that is acceptable to reasonable patient needs under a system of decreased resource availability. Health care leaders have always come through before, and they certainly will do so now.

Appendix A*

The following report was prepared by the Ambulatory Surgery Review Committee of the Health Planning Council, Inc., of Hartford, Connecticut.

Throughout the U.S., many health planning councils and other comprehensive health planning agencies have prepared a great deal of work and effort in evaluating proposals, both within hospitals and within freestanding independently operated facilities, in the area of ambulatory surgery. We have received permission from this particular health planning council to include their report, for which we are very grateful. It is my opinion that the approach taken here is very excellent and can serve as much food-for-thought for other health planning councils, and for health care facilities preparing to embark on a program of ambulatory surgery. We are indebted to Mr. Frederick Margolis, Staff Associate of the Health Planning Council, Inc., in Hartford, Connecticut, for obtaining for us the permission to reprint this report.

---

*Introduction by Thomas R. O'Donovan

185

"The Hartford Report on Ambulatory Surgery"

Testimony to

The Commission on Hospitals
and Health Care

The Hartford Surgical Center, Inc.
Hartford, Connecticut

December 4, 1975

Prepared by:

The Ambulatory Surgery Review
   Committee of the Health
   Planning Council, Inc.

This testimony is submitted to the Commission on Hospitals and Health Care by the Health Planning Council pursuant to its responsibility as an agency under P.L. 89-749, Section 314(b), to review and comment on applications such as the proposed Hartford Surgical Center.

Inasmuch as surgery and surgical facilities had not been researched previously by the Council, a special Ambulatory Surgery Review Committee was established to prepare this testimony. Sufficient data was collected to indicate that adequate resources are available to meet the surgical needs of the region. There is also evidence that less ambulatory surgery is being performed in this region than in other regions which have actively promoted this type of surgery. This is so in spite of the existence of a number of hospital-based ambulatory surgical programs. It was not possible, however, to secure reliable data which would indicate either the factors responsible for the lower comparative rate of ambulatory surgery in the region or the relative differences in cost of developing and operating hospital-based versus freestanding ambulatory surgical programs.

There seems to be general agreement that hospitals should continue developing the capability of doing surgery in the most appropriate setting—inpatient, ambulatory, or outpatient. There is some, but by no means unanimous, opinion that an independent, freestanding ambulatory surgical program should be tried as a possible means of stimulating more surgeons and their patients to accept and use ambulatory surgery in lieu of inpatient surgery.

In view of the lack of adequate information, the committee feels it would be inappropriate for it to make a specific recommendation with respect to the application of the proposed Hartford Surgical Center.

This testimony represents the comments of the Ambulatory Surgery Review Committee as approved by the Health Planning Council Board at its regular noon meeting on November 13, 1975.

A major goal of the Health Planning Council is to facilitate improvement of the health of the residents of its area by promoting programs which should increase the accessibility, acceptability, continuity and quality of the health services provided to the residents, while restraining increases in the costs of providing these health services, preventing unnecessary duplication of health resources, and reducing documented inefficiencies in the area health system. Recent advances in the practice of both surgery and anaesthesiology have led to the development of "ambulatory surgery," a name given to surgery performed under general anaesthesia of sufficiently short duration that the patient can be operated on and discharged all within a period of less than eight hours. These programs hold great potential for increasing the accessibility and acceptability of certain types of surgical procedures while substantially reducing the costs of these procedures to the patient by eliminating the need for overnight confinements in a hospital. The Health Planning Council actively supports ambulatory surgery as an alternative to the more traditional inpatient "overnight" surgical practice, where appropriate, and, consequently, intends to promote the rational development of ambulatory surgery within Health Service Area IV.

The application presently before the Commission on Hospitals and Health Care is a proposal for the development of an ambulatory surgical program and facility by Hartford Surgical Center, Inc. While the Health Planning Council (HPC) recognizes there are numerous potential criteria for evaluating new health care programs, the HPC believes two are of paramount and overriding importance: 1) does there exist a need for the type of service proposed by the applicant; and 2) if such a need exists, will the proposed program fill that need on a quality basis without unduly increasing the overall cost of health care to the community.

The assessment of need for the proposed freestanding surgical center to be located within Health Service Area IV at 100 Retreat Avenue, Hartford requires both an analysis of the need for additional undifferentiated surgical resources, and an analysis of the need for the particular ambulatory surgical resource being proposed.

On the basis of undifferentiated data, this service area appears to have adequate surgical resources now and for the next several years. This absence of need is indicated in a number of ways. First, it is suggested by comparative rates of surgical procedures. Estimates based on data collected by the National Center for Health Statistics indicate a rate of 84.76 inpatient surgical procedures per 1000 population (excluding obstetrical procedures) as the average for the northeastern United States. Presently the number of procedures being performed by the eleven Health Service Area IV hospitals indicate a surgical rate of 85.07 per 1000 population within the area (Table I). The comparable rates suggest that this region's surgical resources are adequate in relation to national and regional experiences.

A stronger indication of the absence of a general need is the existence of eleven unopened operating rooms out of a total of 94 available in area hospitals. These unopened facilities constitute slightly more than eleven percent of the total. Thus, there appears to be considerable capacity to meet present demand and future increases in surgical utilization. In addition, the availability of recovery room beds, as measured by medical/surgical utilization rates, would not appear to constitute limiting factors to performing additional surgical procedures if required (Table II).

Another indicator of the lack of a general need for additional surgical resources, a factor that could act as a constraint on the ability of the regional health system to meet existing and future needs for surgical care, is the availability of surgical personnel. Of particular importance is the availability of general and specialty surgeons. This resource issue does not appear to be a concern in Health Service Area IV at this time. An application of the annual productivity rate for surgical specialists derived by Mason *et al* applied to the surgical specialists (excluding house staff) in practice in Health Service Area IV in 1974 yields an optimal annual output of surgical procedures 26.7 percent

TABLE I

REGIONAL SURGICAL DEMAND ESTIMATES—1975

Population at Risk
HSA Area IV 969,000*

Estimated Number Surgical Operations**	1975	Rate/1000
All Procedures	89,602	
All Procedures Excluding Obstetrical	82,208	84.76
Neurosurgery	1,046	1.08
Ophthalmology	2,757	2.84
Otorhinolaryngology	9,247	9.53
Cardio-vascular Surgery	2,730	2.81
Thoracic Surgery	1,014	1.05
Abdominal Surgery	14,427	14.87
Proctological Surgery	3,012	3.11
Urological Surgery	6,615	6.82
Breast Surgery	2,031	2.10
Gynecological Surgery	16,176	16.68
Obstetrical Procedures	7,394	7.62
Orthopedic Surgery	9,876	10.18
Plastic Surgery	5,217	5.38
Oral and Maxillofacial Surgery	924	.96
Dental Surgery	3,124	3.22
Biopsy	6,012	6.20
Actual Number Surgical Operations		
— all procedures excluding obstetrical	83,063	85.07

* Calculated from 1974 Patient Origin Data from State Health Department population estimates of July 1, 1975.

** Projected from National Center for Health Statistics, "Utilization of Short-Stay Hospitals, Summary of Nonmedical Statistics," 1971.

above actual area demand for 1975. This figure represents a productivity rate for our area surgeons which is 79 percent of the productivity rates derived by Mason. These lower productivity rates appear relatively well-distributed among the various surgical specialties when compared to the rates derived by Mason. Clearly the availability of surgical personnel does not represent a constraining factor on the ability of the area health services system to meet additional demand for surgical procedures (Table III).

TABLE II
SURGICAL RESOURCES IN HOSPITALS IN HSA IV

	Total Number OR's	Number RR Beds	Number SICU Beds	Acute Beds Minus Obs. Beds	Beds Designated for day surgery	Planned Additional OR for ambulatory surgery	Unopened OR units
Hartford Hospital	25	26	12	835	20	2	3 being renovated
St. Francis	19	22	10	525	16		1
Mt. Sinai	10	17	16	291	4		
John Dempsey	4	10	5	59			2
Manchester	6	14	12	239	5		2
New Britain	9	16	19	346			2
Bristol	5[1]	12	2	182			
Bradley	3	6	6	92			1
Rockville	5	10	6	93			
Johnson	3	5	6	66			
Newington	5	8	4	128			
TOTALS	95	146	98	2,856	45	2	11

[1]plus one for minor surgery done with local anaesthetic.

TABLE III
OPTIMAL SURGICAL OUTPUT BY SPECIALTY
HSA REGION IV

	Annual* Productivity Rates	Specialists** HSA Region IV 1974	Optimal Annual Output (Proc.) 1974	Demand*** Estimates 1975	Actual Productivity Rates	% Of Optimal Productivity
General Surgery	282	142	40,044	31,274	220.2	78%
Neurosurgery	113	15	1,695	1,046	69.7	62%
Obstetrical-Gynecological	239	117	27,963	23,570	201.4	84%
Ophthalmology	113	51	5,763	2,757	54.1	48%
Orthopaedics	269	56	15,064	9,876	176.4	65%
Otolaryngology	364	26	9,464	9,247	356.0	98%
Plastic Surgery	264	10	2,640	5,217	521.7	98%
Urology	392	28	10,976	6,615	236.3	60%
All Procedures	255	445	113,609	89,602	201.3	79%

*Derived from Majon, H.R., "Manpower Needs By Specialty," Journal of The American Medical Association, Vol. 219, Mar. 20, 1972, 162-1626.

**Derived from Health Planning Council Inventory of Physicians, 1974.

***Derived from Table I.

If the level of surgical capacity called for in the application (i.e., two operating rooms), regardless of location, is viewed solely as an addition to existing surgical facilities and resources, then it seems clear that no documentable need for the facility exists and that the addition of any undifferentiated surgical resources at this time would be unnecessary duplication.

However, the region's need for the specialized surgical capacities to be provided by the applicant cannot be assessed in terms of undifferentiated need alone. The need for this ambulatory surgical capacity must also be reviewed in terms of existing ambulatory surgical need and the availability of existing resources to meet that need.

Various authors have estimated that, nationally, between 15 and 25 percent of all inpatient surgical procedures could be done safely on an ambulatory surgical basis. Applying those estimates to the current surgical load in the area, the potential number of ambulatory surgical procedures in the greater Hartford region would be between 12,000 and 20,000 surgical procedures a year. This figure constitutes a rate of 13-21 procedures per 1000 population per year. While these estimates of the percentage of surgical procedures appropriate for ambulatory surgery may well be accurate, barriers to the practice of ambulatory surgery exist. Because of these barriers, particularly the present attitudes of some physicians and the attitudes and knowledge of patients, these estimates are useful not as precise estimators of current need, but as overall quantitative targets for optimizing the effectiveness of ambulatory surgical programs in relation to total surgical care in the area.

More immediately useful estimates of need can be derived from the Maricopa County, Arizona utilization experience with ambulatory surgery. After approximately five years experience with ambulatory surgery and substantial increases in ambulatory surgical facilities and programs, both freestanding and hospital-based, the ambulatory surgical rate per 1000 population has grown from 4.7 to approximately 12.6 per 1000 population in Maricopa County. Given the ability of the ambulatory surgical facilities in Maricopa to handle a much larger volume of procedures as evidenced by a utilization rate of the freestanding ambulatory surgical facilities of 52.6 percent, it seems reasonable to utilize the Maricopa County ambulatory surgery rate as a realistic estimate of ambulatory surgical demand which, under optimal conditions, can be generated. It must be noted that certain regional variations in surgical practice exist between Maricopa County, Arizona and this area. However, the Maricopa County ambulatory surgical rate per 1000 population of approximately 12.6 is used in this analysis as the current need estimator for ambulatory surgery for Health Service Area IV.

Presently seven area hospitals are involved in the provision of ambulatory surgery. Certain of these programs are recent in origin and rather limited in scope at the present time; others have been in existence for longer periods and represent larger, more highly organized programs. In Fiscal Year 1975, 6,850 ambulatory surgical procedures were performed in these seven regional hospitals. This represents an ambulatory surgical rate per 1000 population of 7.06 (Table IV). In comparing this rate of ambulatory surgery utilization in Health Service Area IV in Connecticut with the experience of Maricopa County, the ambulatory surgical rate per 1000 population for Maricopa County is approximately 5.0 to 5.8 cases per 1000 population higher than that presently being experienced in Health Service Area IV (Table V). If the Maricopa County experience is taken as a current need estimator, this difference represents an unmet need in ambulatory surgical cases per year of between 4800 and 5600 cases in the greater Hartford region. The Health Planning Council recognizes this need and holds as a priority promoting programs which will reduce the barriers to diminishing this need.

While the total estimated need for ambulatory surgical procedures is not being met currently by the ambulatory surgical programs existing in the area, careful evaluation of the factors involved in the present programs and abilities to meet this need must be investigated before a proper decision is made as to whether the Hartford Surgical Center proposal constitutes unnecessary duplication of ambulatory surgical resources. Certain organizational strengths and shortcomings can be found in both freestanding and hospital-based ambulatory surgical programs.

Specifically, the assessment of whether the Hartford Surgical Center proposal constitutes an unnecessary duplication of the capacity for ambulatory

TABLE IV

AMBULATORY SURGICAL PROCEDURES BY HOSPITAL HSA IV
FY 1975

Hospital	Service* Population	Ambulatory Surgery** Procedures	Rate/1000 pop.
Subarea I			
Bradley Memorial Hospital	19,500	86	4.41
Bristol Hospital	69,800		
New Britain General Hospital	135,300	1,048	7.75
Subarea II			
Hartford Hospital	288,000	2,436	8.46
Mount Sinai Hospital	114,800	154[1]	1.34
St. Francis Hospital	191,100	1,701	8.9
Subarea III			
Dempsey Hospital		7[2]	
Subarea IV			
Manchester Memorial Hospital	103,700	1,418	13.67
Subarea V			
Johnson Memorial Hospital	18,000		
Rockville General Hospital	29,700		
TOTAL	969,900	6,850	7.06

*Calculated from 1974 Patient Origin Data from State Health Department population estimates of July 1, 1975.

**Derived from HPC Ambulatory Surgery Questionnaire.

[1]New program; this figure represents 4 month period from July 1975 to October 1975.

[2]New program; this figiure represents 1 month figures from October 1975.

TABLE V

COMPARISON OF AMBULATORY SURGERY
Maricopa County, Arizona—HSA Region IV, Connecticut

	Maricopa County*	HSA Region IV**
Year	Calendar 1974	FY 1975
Population Estimate	1,350,000	969,900
Ambulatory Surgical Cases Freestanding or Independent Facility	12,073	-0-
Ambulatory Surgical*** Cases Hospital	4,251-5,313	6,850
Total Ambulatory Surgical Cases	16,324-17,386	6,850
Ambulatory Surgery Rate Per 1000 Population	12.09-12.88	7.06
Differential in Ambulatory Surgery Rate Per 1000 Population		5.03-5.82
Differential in Ambulatory Surgery Cases per Year		4,878-5,644
Percent Growth in Utilization From Previous Year	22.6%	15%

*Derived from Comprehensive Health Plan of Maricopa County, 1975.
**Derived from HPC Ambulatory Surgery Questionnaire.
***CHP Council of Maricopa County, Estimate Range based on Arizona Department of Health Services Annual Report.

surgery extant in the region involves the analysis of at least the following factors—the presence or absence of adequate facilities (operating rooms, recovery rooms) for an ambulatory surgery program; the reluctance of some surgeons to perform any or all of their common procedures on an ambulatory surgery basis; the lack of awareness among patients that ambulatory surgery programs exist; and patient reluctance in allowing procedures performed on an ambulatory surgery basis, either because they do not want to ask the surgeon or because they do not feel comfortable with the concept. Thus, the factors equating the demand for ambulatory surgery procedures with the actual need or need estimates for ambulatory surgical procedures can be grouped into two generic categories: 1) inadequacy or unavailability of the physical and programmatic resources required for the provision of the ambulatory surgery; and 2) educational and attitudinal constraints of physicians, surgeons, anaesthesiologists, and patients which inhibit the choice of ambulatory surgery in certain clinical situations.

If, in fact, the major inhibiting factor were inadequacy, unavailability or inaccessibility of facilities or programs for ambulatory surgery, this phenomenon would be represented by certain quantitative characteristics. First, assuming that need surpasses the actual demand for ambulatory surgery and that the changing of attitudinal inhibitions toward ambulatory surgery is a dynamic process based upon both personal and secondary experience, then, given no constraints on the availability, accessibility or adequacy of ambulatory surgical program facilities, the utilization rate or demand for ambulatory surgery should increase at a rate directly proportional to the decrease in the attitudinal inhibitions of the various parties involved. On the other hand, if a facility constraint exists, a static demand rate over time should be observed for ambulatory surgery, or at least, a decrease in the growth rate of ambulatory surgical demand should be observed.

During the past three fiscal years the rate of ambulatory surgery in the region in hospital ambulatory surgery programs has increased. While this growth rate is not as dramatic as that observed in Maricopa County and varies greatly by hospital, it is significant that a small acceleration in rate of increase is present (Table VI).

A second indicator that the differential between the need estimator and the actual ambulatory surgery demand was due to a shortage of available surgical facilities would be a high percentage of ambulatory surgical utilization in relation to operational capacity within each facility.

Presently, the two largest providers of ambulatory services within the region, Hartford Hospital and St. Francis Hospital, have an operational ambulatory surgical capacity of 80 and 60 cases per week, respectively. The latest utilization rates for ambulatory surgery in these two hospitals average 49.3 and 44.5 ambulatory surgery cases per week, respectively, or a net 67 percent utilization rate to operational capacity. Thus, the ambulatory surgical programs of these two hospitals, if running at operational capacity as dictated by demand, could provide under the present administrative arrangements over 2000 additional ambulatory surgical cases per annum.

An additional indication that existing physical facilities were inadequate to the task of meeting present demand or anticipated need would be excessive waiting lists for ambulatory surgical procedures in the area. To test this hypothesis, eight of the most common ambulatory surgical procedures were scheduled hypothetically for day surgery at Hartford Hospital on November 12, 1975 for the first available booking. Table VII shows the first available booking for each procedure and gives the waiting period in days. In five of the

TABLE VI

GROWTH OF AMBULATORY SURGERY IN HSA IV
Number of Ambulatory Surgical Procedures

Hospital	1972-1973	1973-1974	% Change	1974-1975	% Change	Overall % Change 1972-73 to 1974-75
Hartford	1,788	1,882	5%	2,436	30%	36%
St. Francis	1,418	1,647	16%	1,701	3%	20%
Mt. Sinai	0	0	n/a	154	n/a	n/a
John Dempsey	0	0	n/a	7	n/a	n/a
Manchester	1,001	1,338	34%	1,418	6%	42%
New Britain	975	987	1%	1,048	6%	7%
Bradley	53	89	68%	86	-3%	62%
TOTALS	5,235	5,943	14%	6,850	15%	31%
Rate/1000 pop.	5.40	6.13	14%	7.06	15%	31%

TABLE VII

FIRST AVAILABLE DAY SURGERY BOOKING
By Procedure As Of 11-12-75 For Hartford Hospital

Procedure	First Available Booking	Wait in Days
Dilation and Currettage of Uterus, Diagnostic	11-19-75	5
Myringotomy	11-13-75	0
Dental Extraction	11-26-75	10
Breast Biopsy	11-17-75	3
Repair of Inguinal Hernia	11-13-75	0
Sympathectomy of Ganglionec- tomy	11-13-75	0
Augmentation Mammoplasty	11-13-75	0
Blepharoplasty	11-13-75	0

eight procedure categories an opening for day surgery was available on the next day; dental extractions showed the longest waiting period, 10 days. This evidence lends further documentation to the Health Planning Council's conclusion that the differential between need estimates and the actual demand for ambulatory surgery is not attributable in any significant part to actual facility deficiencies, but rather to the attitudinal barriers discussed previously.

The assessment of the appropriateness of a freestanding ambulatory surgical facility and program is difficult given the complexity of the issues and the difficulty in obtaining data pertaining to critical questions. In this testimony we have focused on considerations that we believe to be readily quantifiable to needs and to the possible unnecessary duplication of facilities.

Some controversy exists concerning the relative merits of the ambulatory surgical unit that is hospital-attached and the unit which is independent of such an institution. While the supporters of both types of units maintain that well-organized and properly managed units of either type can provide quality ambulatory surgery effectively, various arguments are raised concerning the preferability of each model.

On the side of the hospital-based programs, it is argued that the immediately available backup potential of the hospital offers greater safety to the patient. Due to the greater availability of inpatient resources, the patient is not placed in jeopardy if a complication develops or if more extensive surgery than originally planned is found to be necessary. Thus, it has been stated that the hospital unit allows the surgeon greater latitude in choosing operative procedures which he is willing to do on an ambulatory basis, due to this added safety factor.

It has also been argued that the range in intensity of surgical procedures (inpatient, ambulatory and outpatient) available in the hospital setting allows for more appropriate utilization of the ambulatory surgery program. While effective screening in either setting can control the performance of inpatient procedures on an ambulatory basis, the availability of outpatient surgical programs in the hospital setting provides a convenient alternative for surgical procedures not requiring general anaesthetic or an intensive recovery period.

The last major advantage cited for the institutional attached unit is that it can be operated more economically than its freestanding counterpart since it avoids duplication of both equipment and staff. While this fiscal saving is not directly observable in lower patient charges it is purportedly significant in reducing community or systems cost.

Supporters of the freestanding setting for ambulatory surgery cite three major advantages to the mode of delivery. First, this type of setting minimizes interference with the doctor-patient relationship by avoiding the fragmentation that often occurs in the larger, more structured hospital environment. The second major advantage of the freestanding type of facility which is cited is the increase in surgeon productivity and decrease in waiting time for elective surgery due to the predictable nature of the procedures performed and proximity of the patient to the operating suite. Lastly, proponents of freestanding facilities claim a saving in cost to the patient when compared to similar procedures performed in hospital-based programs.

Other concerns have been topics of considerable and often involved debate. Perhaps the most notable of these relates to technical quality of services, costs, and provider and consumer satisfaction. A number of concerns in the area of quality were considered by the HPC review committee, including the adequacy of emergency back-up, adequacy of ancillary facilities such as radiological equipment, and safeguards to assure professional competence. The review committee devoted similar attention to issues of costs incurred in providing surgery services in a freestanding setting, in a hospital-based ambulatory surgery program, and under circumstances where the patient is admitted to a hospital as an inpatient. All evidence suggested that charges to the patient are lower when he is operated on within some type of ambulatory surgery program. There have been assertions that considerable savings to the patient may be gained more readily by providing ambulatory surgical services in a freestanding setting than in a hospital-based one.

Given the data presently available, a comparison of costs in the two types of facilities would seem to be invalid for the following reasons: 1) no cost data has been available to date from either type. Selective charges have been furnished but no charge comparisons for the full range of services were made available. Also, no aggregate charges for a standard mix of procedures were available; 2) difference in type of service. Certain services provided in a hospital setting, such as the use of a post recovery bed, are organized somewhat differently than those provided in the proposed Hartford Surgical Center and, therefore, cannot be compared at face value; 3) single pricing. Within each surgical category there are differences in procedural content such as the occasional use of local instead of general anaesthetic which cannot be adequaely discriminated in the single pricing system presented; and 4) charge estimation. The charges cited in the Hartford Surgical Center proposal do not reflect experiential costs but rather estimates which are subject to change. Thus, to make an unequivocal statement about charge comparisons or the total cost to the community of each type of program is impossible at this time. A number of variables, themselves difficult to evaluate with confidence, influence total community cost.

Finally, the committee delved into the questions of professional and patient satisfaction, and again found the issues hazy. With respect to surgeons, for example, members noted that some probably never would feel comfortable performing ambulatory surgery even within a hospital-based program, while others would feel the ambulatory setting, hospital-based or freestanding, was the most appropriate setting for certain procedures. Patients react similarly: some undoubtedly prefer the ready access to the ambulatory setting, particularly that of a freestanding service; others feel secure only as hospital inpatients.

Other questions that were raised which involve qualitative judgments or data which are not at present readily available, are the following:

1) How can the question of need be answered if one considers total regional need vs. the distributed need in specific areas of the region?
2) What is the probability that new facilities will be used by surgeons presently operating the hospital-based ambulatory surgery programs, thus, creating a critical underutilization of extant resources?
3) Will availability of a competitive facility for ambulatory surgery enhance the demand for one-day surgery and keep patient charges at a minimal level?
4) If hospitals direct more operating room time to meet the increasing need for ambulatory surgery, what effect will this have on waiting times for more serious surgery?
5) How much of a factor will public pressure be in changing patterns of demand?
6) From a long range perspective, is it optimal for hospitals to be the institutional setting in which most of the ambulatory surgery is being conducted?
7) How great a factor is the issue of nosocomial infection in recommending that new institutional settings be developed? Can one determine the present rate at a given hospital for ambulatory surgery performed?
8) Are the proposed and actual rates cited in this proposal open to the review process by a public designated agency?
9) Are there other areas of need which should be given greater priority at this time? (e.g., Is the need for facilities in which to perform outpatient surgery under local anaesthesia greater than the need for a facility which would be primarily concerned with ambulatory surgery under general anaesthesia?)

10) What is the cost of opening currently unopened operating rooms, or of constructing additional operating rooms, and how does this compare with the initial costs of the Hartford Surgical Center?

The committee in no way wishes to minimize the importance of these issues or the members' concern for them. Perhaps the key issue concerns the appropriateness of this proposal and other programs in motivating higher utilization of lower cost ambulatory surgery.

The Council feels strongly that the concept of ambulatory surgery must be promoted to the fullest extent possible in our region. Since an optimal review was precluded by insufficient time, data and agreed upon review criteria and standards, the Review Committee was unable to make a clear-cut decision as to whether a freestanding vs. hospital-based ambulatory surgical unit was better for the overall interests of the community. It believes that the data it has developed, which is included as part of this testimony, should be helpful to the Commission in making its decision.

TABLE VIII

NUMBER OF AMBULATORY PROCEDURES CURRENTLY PERFORMED IN HSA IV

Hospital	Total Number of Procedures	Total Ambulatory Surgical Procedures	% Ambulatory Surgical Procedures of Total Surgical Procedures
Hartford Hospital	23,687	2,436	10%
St. Francis	13,154	1,701	13%
Mt. Sinai	10,786	154[1]	6%[3]
John Dempsey	577	7[2]	7%[3]
Manchester	7,349	1,418	19%
New Britain	10,964	1,048	10%
Bristol	6,971	—	—
Bradley	1,492	86	6%
Rockville	2,781	—	—
Johnson	1,102	—	—
Newington	1,442	—	—
TOTALS	80,305	6,850	8.5%

[1]July 1975—October 1975 only.

[2]Month of October 1975 only.

[3]Based on annualized estimates for Mt. Sinai and John Dempsey.

Appendix B

An Evaluation of the Factors that Tend to Differentiate Ambulatory Hospital Surgery from Independently Operated Freestanding Short-Stay Surgical Facilities

Thomas R. O'Donovan

Criteria	In-Hospital Short-Stay Surgery, vs ⟶	Independently Operated Freestanding Ambulatory Care Surgery Facility
1. Cost— To the patient	Probably higher, because of present hospital pricing structure, but the cost could be lower because of the potentially more efficient use of capital by hospitals.	Usually lower
2. Cost— To the community	Probably lower, only if sufficient in-hospital surgical facilities existed in a given area	Probably higher if it duplicates hospital surgical facilities that are not highly utilized

*Reprinted with the permission of Michigan Hospital Association from *Michigan Hospitals,* June 1973.

Criteria	In-Hospital Short-Stay Surgery, vs ⟶	Independently Operated Freestanding Ambulatory Care Surgery Facility
3. Quality of care	Tendency toward being higher, but not in all cases	May be very good, but peer review and other safeguards must be part and parcel of it
4. Access to care a) If hospital facilities are at total capacity in the local area	Restrictive	Would increase access by providing for much needed additional facilities (depending on how carefully placed they were)
(b) If hospital facilities are not at total capacity	Then access is not aided by duplicating services	No increase in access
(c) If patients lack ability to pay	The non-profit community hospital tends to render care based more on need of care than on ability to pay; hence access to care is increased in those instances.	Depends on the individual situation
5. Continuity of care	Tendency toward increase	A decrease, but this isn't the purpose of come and go surgery
6. Comprehensiveness of care	Tendency toward increase	A decrease, but this isn't the purpose of come and go surgery
7. Patient satisfaction	Reduce; hospital admission policies are often bureaucratic and inefficient, but this could certainly be improved; other areas besides admission policies must be evaluated, however	Tendency toward increase, especially if admission procedures are highly streamlined and efficient. The Phoenix Surgicenter® certainly has provided a national bulwark of excellence in this criteria

Criteria	In-Hospital Short-Stay Surgery, vs ⟶	Independently Operated Freestanding Ambulatory Care Surgery Facility
8. Framentation of the health care delivery system	Tendency toward low fragmentation	In a first-rate facility, such as the Phoenix Surgicenter,® there may be a consolidation because a better division of labor may be provided
9. Dynamics of responsiveness to changing community needs	The freestanding advocates claim that hospitals are too bureaucratic to be highly responsive; however, many hospitals may respond well because they may be able to detect needs quickly due to its great community contact and broad range of services	Possibly greater, depending on how well they are managed

Appendix C

Common Operative Procedures in Ambulatory Surgery— A Master Listing

---

Aristospan injection
Arthrodesis (phalanges) (Other joints)
Arthroplasty (phalanges) (Other joints)
Arthroscopy
Arthrotomy, meniscetomy
Adhesions of clitoris
Abscess, I & D
A-V fistula
Adenoidectomy and Myringotomy
Arch Bars, removal or application
Aspiration of Aqueous
Augmentation mammoplasty (unilateral) (bilateral)

Bartholin cystectomy
Biopsy-vulva
Bone graft
Bone reconstruction
Bunion operation
Bursae, removal of (olecranon)

Biopsy, conjunctiva or cornea
Benign Intraoral lesions
Branchial arch appendages, excision
Basal cell CA, excision
Blepharoplasty (upper or lower or combined)
Biopsy liver
Bone marrow biopsy
Brachial clefts
Breast implant, removal
Breat masses, excision
Bronchoscopy

Carpal tunnel decompression
Carpal tunnel ligament release
Cast change with manipulation
Cervical node biopsy
Colonoscopy
Cataract—by phakoemulsification
Curettage or cauterization of corneal ulcer
Chalazion

Cryoretinopexy
Culdocentesis
Carbuncle, excision
Circumcision
Cystoscopy
Canthus excision
Cryopexy for retinal tear
Cyst excision
Cardioversion
Cryotherapy, alone
Caudal
Celiac (Splanchnic)
Cleft lip repair
Capsulectomy
Closed reduction (nose or zygoma)
Correction hammer toe (Repair and plastic operation joints of foot and toes)
Colostomy, revision
Cautery vaginal cyst
Cervical amputation (sturmdorf)
Cervical cone
Colpotomy, diagnostic
Cryotherapy (alone)
Cryotherapy (with biopsy)
Culdoscopy
Culdocentesis
Cystectomy-Skene's Duct

Dermabrasion (partial or full)
Dessication of condyloma
Dorsal slit
Debridement
Dislocated shoulder or elbow
Dermoid cyst of eyebrow, excision
Discission
Dilation and curettage

Episiotomy
Electroschock therapy
Exostosis, excision
Examination under anesthesia

Excision of Urethral Caruncle
Ectropion and entropion
Enucleation
Eye muscle operation—recession (unilateral)
Exostosis, Excision
Esophagoscopy
Excision, foreign bodies
Excision, lesions, skin tags, cysts
Excisions of parotid and submaxillary stones
Ethmoidectomy
Excision of skin tumors (local vs. wide or radical-Wilz)
Esophageal dilatation

Fissure in ano
Fistula in ano
Fistulectomy
Foreign body, removal (with or without x-ray)
Frenulectomy, tongue—in children
Fracture, closed reduction, uncomplicated
Fracture, closed reduction (with or without x-ray)
Fundoscopic exam in children
Facial wire, removal
Flap revision
Facila and neck lesions
Fulguration of bladder neck
Fasciectomy (finger) (palm)
Foreign body excision
Foreign body excision, with x-ray
Foreign body removal, ear
Fusion

Gastroscopy
Gynecomastia, excision
Ganglionectomy

Hair Transplantations

Hymenotomy
Hysteroscopy
Hydrocelectomy
Hand infections (minor and major)
Hemangioma, removal
Hemorrhoidectomy
Hemorrhoidectomy, thrombotic
Herniorrhaphy, inguinal (infant or adult—unilateral or bilateral)
Herniorrhaphy, unbilical
Hand fasciectomy for arthritis
Hammertoes with tenotomies and resection of bones
Hardware, removal
Hardware, removal, hip
Hemangioma, nostril

Injection of intervertebral disc
Inferior Turbinate Fracture
Intercostal neurectomy
Inclusion cyst, excision
Inferior turbinate fracture
Inguinal/scrotal abscess, I and D
Iridectomy
Intercostal
Impacted wisdom teeth, removal of
Incision & drainage dental
Intra-oral Biopsy

Jaw, wiring of

Kidney cannula, revision
Keratotomy
Kordiolum

Litholapaxy (Bladder stone crusing & removal)
Laparoscopy
Lipoma, excision
Lacrimal duct probing or reconstruction
Laryngoscopy
Labia lesion, excision

Laryngeal polypectomy
Laryngoscopy with operative procedure
Limited Rhinoplasty
Lymph Node Biopsy
Lesion excision with graft
Limited chemical face peel
Limited face lifts
Limited septo-rhinoplasty
Lipectomy

Myringoplasty
Meloplasty
Muscle biopsy
Meatotomy
Minor Salivary Gland Surgery
Multiple teeth extractions
Myotomy—recession or resection
Manipulation of joints (with or without x-ray)
Mass excision with scar revision
Medial ligament, knee, repair of
Metatarsal heads, excision
Morton's neuroma
Mastoidectomy
Mouth biopsy
Myringotomy with or without tubes
Mammoplasty, augmentation or revision

Nasal fractures
Nasal polyp, removal
Nose, closed fracture reduction
Nerve repair
Neuroma (other)
Neurolysis (finger)

Orchiectomy
Orchiopexy
Odontectomy, uncomplicated
Odontectomy, surgical
Oral surgery
Olecranon spur, excision

Olecranon bursa, excision
Olecranon spur, excision
Open reduction fracture, without x-ray
Osteotomy
Odontectomy, surgical
Otoscopy
Otoscopy (with removal foreign body)
Open and closed zygomatic fractures
Otoplasty

Perineorrhaphy
Polypectomy, cervical
Periodontic surgery (full or partial)
Photocoagulation
Pterygium
Phalangectomy
Planter wart, excision
Pedicle flap, transfer
Paracentesis
Pilonidal cystectomy
Prostate biopsy
Pelvic encoscopy (Schirodkar)
Palate biopsy
Poly tubes, removal
Preauricular cyst excision
Periodontal surgery
Placement dental arches
Pre-prosthesis surgery

Rectal biopsy
Rhinoplasty
Rhytidoplasty
Resection (unilateral)
Resection (bilateral)
Removal Mandibular/Maxillary Cyst
Removal soft tissue tumors
Reduction of minor facial fractures
Reduction of nasal fractures
Rhytidectomy with blepharoplasty

Renal biopsy

Scalene node biopsy
Skin lesions, excision
Spinal tap
Septal reconstruction
Strabotomy, pediatric
Scar revisions and relaxations
Skin grafts, minor
Sequestrectomy
Synovectomy
Saline injection, intrauterine-therapeutic
Sturmdorf repair of cervix
Stapedectomy
Submucous resection
Simple tendon repairs
Surgical correction of prominent ear
Sub-dural tap
Splanchnic (Celiac)
Stellate

Thyroglossal duct cyst
Tendon repair
Tenosynovectomy
Tenotomy, hand or foot
Trigger finger release
Tonsillectomy, with or without adenoidectomy
Tarsorrhaphy
Therapeutic retrobulbar injections
Thoracentesis, closed
Torticollis, repair
Therapeutic abortion
Trans-vaginal ligation of tubes
Tubal coagulation or ligation
Tension measurements in children
Tongue biopsy
Tongue surgery-glossectomy
Tonsillar tag excision
Tympanoplasty
Testes, excision
Testicular biopsy

Testicular prosthesis insertion

Urethral dilation—in children
Urethroscopy—in children
Ulnar nerve transfer
Urethral catheter
Umbilical herniorrhaphy with
    bilateral inguinal herniorrhaphy
Umbilical sinus, excision

Vulva biopsy
Vasectomy
Vasograms
Varicocelectomy
Varicose vein ligation

Varicotomy
Vaginal stenosis, release
Vaginal tumor, excision
Vaginal web, excision
Vaginoplasty
Ventral femoral hernia
Vermillionectomy (upper or lower
    lip)
Vermillionectomy (both lips)

Xanthoma, excision

Z-plasty
Zygomatic arch
Zygoma, reduction

Appendix D
Patient Information Booklets

Following is an example of a "patient information booklet" that any health care facility can use as a partial model for their own program of ambulatory surgery.

"AMBULATORY SURGERY"

Surgery Without Hospitalization

Modern medical advances now make it possible, in many instances, for patients to receive surgical treatment under complete hospital conditions—and return to their homes, all in the same day.

The Out-Patient Surgical Center was created for just such circumstances—to serve patients who need surgical treatment exceeding the capability of the usual physician's office but for whom overnight hospitalization is not anticipated. Establishment of this specialized facility helps us move toward two continuing objectives, reduced cost to patients and increased effectiveness in the utilization of hospital facilities.

For the patient, in addition to the materially lower hospital bill, elimination of an extended period of separation from home and family can have many beneficial results. And, although the Out-Patient Surgical Center is designed to be completely self-sufficient in its specialized function, the facilities of a complete hospital are immediately available should circumstances require.

Besides eliminating the cost of overnight care and capabilities associated with round-the-clock activities, other steps have been taken to minimize administrative and overhead costs. To simplify accounting, an inclusive hospital fee is charged for the use of the facility—varying according to the surgical procedure involved.

This inclusive charge covers use of the operating room and all equipment, routine laboratory work, recovery room, all drugs and medicines administered and preparation of all appropriate reports and records.

Fees for professional services (your physician, surgeon and assistants, radiologists, anesthesiologists) are not included in this inclusive hospital charge.

Admitting Procedures

As a patient, you will be scheduled into the Out-Patient Surgical Center by your own attending physician. If he anticipates need for another surgeon or for an anesthesiologist, pathologist or similar medical specialist, he will make the necessary arrangements. Your physician will advise you regarding the time your surgery is scheduled.

If your surgery is scheduled a week or more in advance, a pre-admission form will be mailed to you by the hospital. The amount of your hospital charge will be noted on this pre-admit form. We request that you remit this amount if you do not have applicable insurance—or $35 and the group insurance forms if you are covered. Please mail your payment and forms to us at least four days prior to your scheduled surgery.

If your surgery is scheduled in less than a week, you will be contacted by telephone. Please give the person contacting you the pre-admit information and bring your payment and insurance forms with you when you come for surgery.

Patients should come to the OPS reception room 45 minutes prior to their surgery time and report to the admitting secretary. Necessary consent forms, medical history, pre-operative evaluation, laboratory work and administrative procedures will be completed at this time, unless this has been done previously. In the case of minors, the consent form must be signed by a parent or guardian.

Casual clothing that can be folded and stored during your operation is most convenient. Robe and slippers and the surgical gown will be furnished at the OPS.

Patients should not eat or drink anything after midnight on the day of their operation and should eat only lightly on the evening before. This is extremely important for patient safety.

Jewelry and valuables—including watches—should be left at home. If you wear glasses or dentures you may want them during waiting and post-recovery periods.

It is important that you arrange to have someone drive you home. Patients cannot be permitted to leave alone after an operation. Your physician will be able to estimate the hour when you will be able to go home so that you may make necessary arrangements. If your driver waits for you, reading material is obtainable in the hospital pharmacy, and the facilities of the coffee shop and hospital cafeteria are available.

Important Post-Operative Instructions

When you have returned home, be sure to follow your physician's instructions regarding rest, medication and diet.

Unless given other directions, drink only clear liquids for the first six hours after your operation. Then, if you are comfortable with the liquids, you may add progressively to your diet according to your doctor's instructions. You should not drink alcoholic beverages until 24 hours after anesthesia.

It is normal to feel a little dizzy and sleepy after an operation. Therefore, you must not drive or operate machinery for at least 12 hours. Nor should you make important decisions or sign important papers until this feeling has worn off.

Out-Patient Treatment Program

The Out-Patient Surgical Center is part of an expanding program to provide an increasing variety of medical services, when appropriate, on an out-patient basis. Besides the obvious financial savings for patients, in many instances there are other personal and psychological benefits that can speed recovery, reduce worry and apprehension, and minimize family and home disruption.

Equally important, perhaps, the out-patient programs extend the availability of our Hospital's facilities to a greater number of people in the community, reserve our hospital-bed capacity for those who must be hospitalized, and multiply the impact of the philanthropy of many generous donors whose gifts have built this hospital.

To make this out-patient program most effective, we welcome reactions and recommendations from those who have participated in it. In your follow-up contacts after your operation, we urge you to give us the benefit of your comments.

A GUIDE FOR PATIENTS FOR AMBULATORY SURGERY

Pre-Admission

As preparation for your procedure your doctor may have given instructions for x-ray, laboratory and other tests. Your doctor will complete a history and physical sheet and your surgeon will have you sign an Operative Consent Form prior to your admission to the Short Procedures Unit.

You have an appointment in the Short Procedures Unit on _____ at _____ for these tests.
           (date)   (time)

An interview with a physician from the Anesthesia Department has also been scheduled for you at this time.

It is imperative that you notify the Short Procedures Unit 24 hours in advance if you can not keep this appointment.

Admission

Please come to the Short Procedures Unit on _____
(date)

at _____ (This is one (1) hour before your scheduled operat-
       (time)
ing room time.)

1. Please have nothing to eat or drink after midnight the night before surgery. Failure to comply with this request could result in a cancellation of your procedure.
2. Please leave valuables and jewelry at home. Make-up and nail polish should not be worn. We are not responsible for lost or stolen articles.
3. Because you may be drowsy for some time following your procedure, you MUST BE ACCOMPANIED BY A DRIVER. Persons accompanying you to and from the hospital may wait in the Family Lounge on the first floor of the Highland Wing.

Discharge

You are discharged from the Short Procedures Unit on order of your doctor. Please plan on an average stay of four (4) hours if you are to receive general anesthesia.

Financial Policy

Short Procedures Unit costs, including pre-admission testing, are outpatient charges which are due and payable at the time service is provided. Charges for use of the Unit are based on an hourly rate, plus charges for operating room, anesthesiology, and other ancillary services.

The Registrar will review with you your insurance coverages and required authorization prior to admission. Patients having private insurance (not Blue Cross or Intercounty) are expected to pay their bills in full and arrange for their own reimbursements. Charges are to be paid at Registrar's desk.

Objective

The Short Procedures Unit, one of the first to be established in this area, is recognized as an effective alternative to expensive, time-consuming inpatient stays. Your physician has determined that your procedure does not require an overnight stay in the hospital; thus you avoid using a bed needed for more seriously ill patients.

Finally

The Short Procedures Unit is designed for the best utilization of all facilities contained in your community hospital. Your suggestions are welcome.

Appendix E

Forms Used in
Ambulatory Surgery

PRE-ADMISSION AND SHORT PROCEDURES RESERVATION

DATE RESERVATION MADE _____ BY WHOM _____

PATIENT NAME *(last name first)*_____

DATE OF BIRTH *(Mo. Date Yr.)*_____ SEX_____ RACE_____ AGE_____

ADDRESS _____ CITY _____ STATE_____ ZIP _____

TELEPHONE NUMBER _____ SERVICE DR._____

DIAGNOSIS _____

PROCEDURE OR TREATMENT_____

PRE-OPERATIVE ORDERS _____

CONSULTATIONS _____

ANESTHESIA_____

LISTED BELOW ARE THE TESTS OR STUDIES REQUIRED PRIOR TO ADMISSION TO
THE SHORT PROCEDURES UNIT OR TO THE HOSPITAL.

SCHEDULES DATE_____

_____   _____   _____

_____   _____   _____

_____   _____   _____

HAVE HISTORY AND PHYSICAL FORM AND CONSENT FORM BEEN COMPLETED?

YES ☐   NO ☐

WHEN WILL THEY BE RECEIVED _____
DATE SCHEDULED FOR PROCEDURE _____
TIME SCHEDULED FOR O.R._____
DATE THAT PATIENT WAS CALLED_____
TIME PATIENT DUE IN UNIT _____

ADMITTED TO UNIT	DISCHARGED FROM UNIT	SUB TOTAL	SENT TO O.R.	RETURNED FROM O.R.	SUB TOTAL	TOTAL HOURS	COST

RESPONSIBLE PARTY _____

ADDRESS _____ CITY _____ STATE____ ZIP ____

TELEPHONE NUMBER _____ INSURANCE_____

TYPE OF CONTRACT _____ GROUP NUMBER_____

CERTIFICATE NUMBER _____ EFFECTIVE DATE_____

COMMENTS_____

PRESBYTERIAN HOSPITAL OF DALLAS

CONSENT TO OPERATION

Patient:_____ Age:_____

A.M.

Date:_____ Time:_____P.M. Place:_____

1. I hereby authorize Dr. _____ and
    whomever he may designate as his assistants, to perform upon

    _____ the following operation:
    (state name of patient or "myself")

    _____:
    (state nature of procedure(s) to be performed)

    and if any unforeseen condition arises in the course of the operation calling
    on his judgment for procedures in addition to or different from those now
    contemplated, I further request and authorize him to do whatever he
    deems advisable.

2. The nature and purpose of the operation, possible alternative methods of treatment, the risks involved, and the possibility of complications have been fully explained to me. I acknowledge that no guarantee or assurance has been made as to the results that may be obtained.

3. I consent to the administration of anesthesia to be applied by or under the direction of Dr. _____
and to the use of such anesthetics as he may deem advisable.

I certify that I have read and fully understand the above consent to operation, that the explanations therein referred to were made, and that all blanks or statements requiring insertion or completion were filled in before I affixed my signature.

Signed: _____
(Patient or person authorized to consent for patient)

Witness: _____

Witness: _____

PRESBYTERIAN HOSPITAL OF DALLAS

FATHER'S CONSENT FOR SURGERY ON MINOR

TO: Doctor _____
at the Presbyterian Hospital of Dallas:

The undersigned having requested that you perform an operation on a minor child, viz: _____,
this is your full and unconditional authority to proceed with anesthetics, surgery, diagnosis and treatment as your judgment indicates; further, if in the course of the contemplated operation a different, or more extensive operation in your judgment is required, you are fully authorized to proceed therewith, and it is distinctly agreed and understood that you and your associates as physi-

cians and surgeons shall not be responsible in any way for any consequences resulting from said operation, anesthetics, diagnosis and treatment, and you and each of you are hereby fully released from any and all claims and demands whatsoever which might arise, grow out of or be incident to such diagnosis, operation or treatment, and the undersigned is obligated and bound to hold you and your associates harmless from any and all consequences for such treatment, diagnosis or surgery, provided that your duties are performed with ordinary care and to the best of your ability.

WITNESS MY HAND THIS_____day of_____, A.D. 19_____.

Signed: _____
                     (Father)   (Mother*)

WITNESS: _____

WITNESS: _____

*This consent is given by me as mother of said child because my husband is not available to specifically authorize the procedure at this time, although he is cognizant of the child's condition and believes as I do, that such operation is necessary for the welfare of said child.

PRESBYTERIAN HOSPITAL OF DALLAS

INFORMATION SHEET FOR
DAY SURGERY PATIENTS

Your surgery is scheduled for_____a.m. on _____.
                                               (time)   (date)
Report to the Day Surgery Unit at_____ a.m.
                                                        (time)
the day of scheduled surgery. If you are unfamiliar with the location of the Day Surgery Unit, please ask for assistance at the front lobby Information Desk.

Important Facts to Remember:

(1) *DO NOT EAT OR DRINK ANYTHING AFTER THE MIDNIGHT BEFORE SURGERY!*

(2) When coming to the Hospital for pre-admission procedures and on the day of scheduled surgery, park your car in the front Visitors Parking Lot.

(3) A member of your family or a friend may remain with you in your room throughout the day of your surgery. *Visitors are limited to one* and they must be fourteen years of age or older.

(4) Leave your valuables at home or give them to a family member for safekeeping.

(5) Please bring a robe and slippers. Since your stay will be a short one, it is not necessary to bring many personal items.

(6) It will be necessary that you make arrangements in advance for transportation home so that when your physician discharges you, you will not be delayed.

(7) Upon discharge, you or a member of your family, will be escorted to the Business Office for financial out-processing, and then you will be taken to the Emergency Room entrance where the individual accompanying you will pick you up.

(8) No food trays are served in the Day Surgery Unit and no food is allowed in this Unit from the Cafeteria or the Coffee Shop.

(9) Flowers are not delivered to the Day Surgery Unit due to the short duration of stay and the lack of space.

(10) Public telephones are available for your use and are located in the Surgery-Family Waiting Room opposite the Physical Medicine Department on the Lower Level.

We are looking forward to your visit and hope your stay will be a pleasant one.

BAPTIST MEDICAL CENTER OUTPATIENT SURGERY

No. ____

DATE / /

PATIENT'S NAME (LAST) (FIRST) (MIDDLE)   AGE   DATE OF BIRTH   SURGEON

ADDRESS   CITY   STATE   ZIP CODE   PHONE   RACE   MARITAL STATUS   S   M   SEP.   W   D

RESPONSIBLE PARTY NAME   ADDRESS   CITY   STATE   ZIP CODE   TELEPHONE

EMPLOYER NAME   EMPLOYER ADDRESS   SOC. SEC. NO.

INSURANCE CO.   GROUP NO.   SUBSCRIBER NO.   UNDER NAME OF   IN PLAN AT CITY   OTHER INSURANCE

CHARGE:

ADMITTING DIAGNOSIS   OPERATION PERFORMED

LABORATORY
URINALYSIS   RH   HCT   WBC   PTT   RPR   VITAL SIGNS   B/P   PULSE   HEIGHT   WEIGHT   ALLERGIES
TEMP.

HISTORY: ✓ NO ABNORMALITY   X ABNORMALITY (DESCRIBE)
BLEEDING TENDENCIES   STEROIDS   DIABETES   TB   HEENT   G.I.   G.U.

NEURO-MUSCULAR   EXTREMITIES   GENITALIA   PREVIOUS SURG.   MEDICATIONS

PRE-OPERATIVE MEDICAL EXAMINATION & STATUS OF HEART & LUNGS

NPO SINCE   DENTURES   CONT. LENS   PRE-OPERATIVE MEDICATIONS

GEN. [ ]   LOC [ ]   BLK [ ]   INTUB. YES [ ] NO [ ]   I.V. FLUIDS:

POST - OP ORDERS:

BARBIT.   160
N₂O   140
O₂   120
FLUO   100
RELAXANT   80
         60
XYLOCAINE   40
         20

DETAILS OF
ANESTHESIA
OTHER REMARKS

OPERATION TIME   TO   ANESTHESIA TIME   TO   DRAINS   SPONGE COUNT   SPECIMEN - DISPOSITION

X-RAY   E.B.L.   CIRCULATING NURSE   SCRUB NURSE

OPERATIVE REPORT:

SIGNATURE OF ANESTHESIOLOGIST

SIGNATURE OF SURGEON

DATE

RECOVERY ROOM – POST OP COURSE

TIME RECEIVED | AM PM | COMMENTS:

160
140
120
100
80
60
40
20

TIME RELEASED | A.M. P.M. | RELEASED TO WHOM

MEDICAL RECORDS

5954 12-75

BAPTIST MEDICAL CENTER OUTPATIENT SURGERY

COMPLICATION FOLLOW-UP

PATIENT'S NAME: _____ TELEPHONE NUMBER: _____

OPERATIVE PROCEDURE: _____

DATE OF SURGERY: _____ SURGEON: _____

NURSE _____

Appendix F
Suggested Equipment for Ambulatory Surgery Services*

Operating Room Area

Fixed equipment, each operating room:
- Isolation transformer, monitor, circuitry
- Ground outlets and cables
- Ceiling mounted surgical light with wall-mounted, intensity controls
- X-ray view box, wall-flush mounted
- Gas alarms, shut-off valves, gauges for pressures and reserve line indicators (latter if required)
- Availability of oxygen, nitrogen, nitrous oxide, and suction
- Communication system flush-wall mounted

Major moveable equipment for each operating room:
- General operating table and facilities for storage of parts
- Stools for the surgeon and the anesthesiologist
- Instrument and pack tables
- Cautery machines with cabinet for parts
- Anesthesia machine with scavenger device and mounted battery operated monitor

Portable and fragile equipment for a multi-procedure operating room (requires separate in-suite storage space for protection when not in use):
- Crash cart with mounted monitor and defibrillator
- Operating microscope and cabinets for microscopes and lens
- Laparoscopy equipment with cabinets
- Bronchoscopy and laryngoscopy equipment with battery boxes and carts for scopes

*From the Ambulatory Surgery Criteria and Standards Monograph prepared by Marie Erbstoeszer, University of Washington, for The Health Resources Administration, Department of Health, Education, and Welfare, Contract No. HRA 106-74-56, 1975.

- Portable x-ray machine, cassettes, and film
- Urology and/or orthopedic tables
- Lead aprons and gloves
- Drills (oral, orthopedic, dental)
- Cast cart, orthopedic equipment and materials
- Aspirator for termination of pregnancy, if performed
- Pneumatic tourniquets, regulators, and insufflators
- Anesthesia ventilator and positive pressure machines
- Ophthalmological equipment with related cylinders and parts cabinet
- Cystoscopic equipment, parts cabinets, and battery boxes
- Portable oxygen and suction equipment

Decontaminating Area

- Triple sinks with wall mounted faucets for cleaning lumens
- Flush sink with plaster trap
- Communication system
- Wall mounted peg board for draining of hoses
- Closed hampers for soiled materials

Autoclave Area

Fixed equipment:
- Hi vacuum sterilizer and general steam sterilizer
- Autoclave cart loaders
- Carts for "cold" sterilization of scopes

Pharmacy Area

- Work shelving
- Locked storage cabinets
- Solutions storage
- Drug refrigerator
- Hand wash sink
- Records control desk

Appendix G
An Answer to Soaring Hospital Costs?*

One-day Surgery Could Improve—or Maybe Wreck—the Health-Care System

James Felske, 6, recently had his tonsils and adenoids removed at Northwest Surgicare in Arlington Heights, Ill., at a cost of $169—about a third of the $480 charged by most Chicago area hospitals. Yet Northwest Surgicare is no charity insitution. On the contrary, it is an example of a controversial new kind of profit-making business: an ambulatory surgical facility (ASF), where doctors perform simple operations that do not require an overnight stay. James's bill included neither the room-and-bed charges of a conventional hospital nor the overhead cost of maintaining expensive hospital equipment for treatment more serious than his. Moreover, no hospital—with its set routine and focus on life-and-death cases—could have given James the personal attention he received.

But James's gain may be the hospitals' loss, with drastic effects on the life-and-death cases. If such patients do not help pay for the hospital's dialysis machine, emergency room, and 24-hour nursing service, asks hospital industry spokesmen, what happens to the patient who needs them?

The $548 that Chicago's Michael Reese Hospital charges for a tonsillectomy—certainly more than its direct cost—subsidizes far more complex operations. Hospital spokesmen ask: How can hospitals, already in dire financial straits, continue to serve the community if ASFs strip them of their only "profitable" business?

"This could be the hottest issue in the health care field," said one participant in a recent conference on ASFs.

---

*Reprinted from the July 7, 1975 issue of *Business Week* by special permission. © 1975 by McGraw-Hill, Inc.

225

The typical ambulatory surgical facility has two or more operating rooms, a recovery area, and emergency backup arrangements with a nearby hospital. It is equipped to do some 125 low-risk operations on healthy, low-risk patients. The patient comes in, undergoes tests and surgery, rests, and goes home—all in one day.

Savings. To its backers, the case for the new industry is overwhelming. They contend that ambulatory surgical facilities could transform the U.S. health care system by reducing the cost and humanizing the conditions of minor surgery, a category that covers at least a third of all hospital operations.

Such a switch would lop an estimated $6-billion to $15-billion off the nation's $115-billion health-care bill, generating spectacular savings for both health insurance companies and the employers and consumers who pay their premiums. Metropolitan Life Insurance Co., which honors claims from 22 ASFs under group health insurance policies, figures that it has saved $1-million in the five years since Surgicenter, the first such facility, opened in Phoenix.

No one seems to know how many have opened since then. Estimates range from 24—from Surgicenter cofounder Dr. Wallace Reed, who is also president of the newly formed Society for the Advancement of Free-Standing Ambulatory Surgical Care (SAFSASC)—to close to 100—from Joseph H. Clune, manager of Metropolitan Life's group claims division, whose personal certification of new units for company coverage has made him an authority on the subject. Whatever the total, everyone agrees that it is rising fast.

"ASFs have to grow as long as hospital prices keep going up," says Clune. "We're for it, provided they observe strict professional standards. We're for anything in the way of good hospital care that will cut our costs."

Government study. Apparently the government shares his view. The Social Security Administration has contracted for a study by Orkand Corp., a health-planning research agency, to determine whether ambulatory surgical facilities should qualify for medicare reimbursement—a decision that would give the new industry a significant extra push.

The ASFs already in business vary widely, from modest units to the $3.5-million Bailey Square Surgical Center in Austin, Tex., with seven operating rooms. Doctors use them like hospitals, paying no fee, and billing the patient separately. ASFs are always bargains. Riffling through Metropolitan Life's files, Clune notes such contrasting average charges as $435 for removal of a breast tumor in a hospital compared with $131 in an ASF.

Most ambulatory surgical facilities start making money after two years. Northwest Surgicare, currently averaging 55 operations a week in four operating rooms, projects an eventual annual return of 10% to 15% for the 17 doctors who invested $350,000 in the project. Other ASF operators regard 20% as a reasonable return.

Hospital opposition. But all is not roses along this road to reduced patient costs and increased investor profits. Skimming off low-risk, no-overhead surgery from hospitals will simply increase the cost of those operations that must be performed in hospitals, says Dr. Herbert Notkin, former director of the American Hospital Assn.'s ambulatory care division. And Dr. Peter Rogatz, senior vice-president of Blue Cross-Blue Shield of Greater New York, stresses that increased ambulatory surgical care will aggravate the problem of surplus hospital beds.

"Ambulatory surgery has got to be less expensive, nobody is going to disagree with that. But we can't develop this as a viable system of health care delivery unless we also deal with the over-bedding problem," Rogatz says. "In other words, close hospitals."

Trying to close hospitals, however, provokes violent objections from both inner-city residents, whose hospitals often provide their only source of health care, and suburbanites, who regard local hospitals as local amenities. Hospital trustees and administrators also frequently resist closing "their" hospitals, empty beds or not.

As a result, say backers of the new concept, hospital groups have attacked ambulatory centers as medically unsound or unnecessary, throwing up legal barriers through their political influence on regional health-planning agencies. The backers distinguish emphatically between these restrictions and the quality controls they concede are needed because of the lack of formal accreditation procedures. The industry group is working up recommendations for qualifications to present to a society meeting in November.

To the AHA, this lack, with its appeal to quick-buck operators, constitutes the crucial difference between the 2,300 hospital-linked ambulatory surgical units and the independent ones. The hospital association has encouraged such care since the first unit opened 15 years ago in Watts Hospital in Durham, N.C., says AHA President John A. McMahon. Other officials insist that busy hospitals actually support all responsible ambulatory centers, hospital-linked or profit-making, to free their equipment for the seriously ill.

But not all hospitals are busy, and those that are not are ready to fight fiercely anything that could empty still more beds. "In a lot of hospitals," says Metropolitan Life's Clune, "Saturday is tonsillectomy day."

Moreover, the hospital-affiliated ambulatory surgical care unit cannot really compete with the independent on price because it bears some of the hospital's overhead costs. If James Felske had had his tonsillectomy at Michael Reese's ambulatory unit, his bill would have been $381—more than twice Northwest Surgicare's price and only a third less than the bill for an inpatient tonsillectomy at Michael Reese.

Showing compassion. To the ASF patient, however, price seems to matter less than atmosphere. "Almost nobody comes here because it's cheaper," says Dr. Herbert E. Natof, medical director of Northwest Surgicare "The insurance is going to pay for it anyway. The patient comes because he wants to avoid the impersonal, inconvenient treatment he associates with hospitals. We're small, we deal with a few people at a time, and we really work hard at treating people kindly."

Dr. M. Robert Knapp, co-founder of the Minor Surgery Center in Wichita, Kan., sums up the case for ASFs: "Due to their small size and very limited function, free-standing ambulatory surgical facilities will always be able to deliver better service at a lower cost than larger health-care institutions," he says. They save money, says Knapp, and they also treat patients with compassion. To which a hospital official might reply: "What about the patient who needs dialysis more than he needs compassion?"

Appendix H

Ambulatory Surgery at Mt. Carmel Mercy Hospital: Excellent Service to Patients*

A hospitalization, even for one familiar with hospital procedures, is a stressful event for a patient. Under the most comfortable of circumstances it requires adjustment to unfamiliar and sometimes unnerving surroundings, disrupts family routine, and in diverse ways is a costly event.

Growing out of some of these reasons—and many more—a new approach to patient surgical procedures, with a minimum of time spent in the hospital, is the rapidly developing program in major hospitals across the country of Ambulatory Surgery—or Short-Stay Surgery, as it is sometimes also called.

At Mount Carmel Mercy Hospital and Medical Center, Ambulatory Surgery was initiated in an investigative way in 1974, and during the past year a full-fledged acceptance has been increasingly utilized as a modern approach to patient care. As more and more physicians are taking advantage of the program and the facilities in the new North Tower surgical suite, it is becoming clearer, how the patient benefits, the hospital benefits by freeing more beds for the care of acutely ill patients, and the physician benefits in being able to reserve more time for the more seriously ill.

Mount Carmel began an Ambulatory Surgery program in 1974 when 117 patients were scheduled for this one-day type of procedure. In 1975, that number jumped dramatically to 1,246 patients, and the total is expected to increase greatly again in 1976. Nationally, it is a mushrooming concept of hospital service.

---

*From *Mount Carmel Reflector,* February, 1976, pp. 6-7. (Mount Carmel Mercy Hospital and Medical Center, Detroit, Michigan).

As Dr. Willard S. Holt, chairman of Mount Carmel's Ambulatory Surgery Department, says, "At Mount Carmel, we haven't jumped right in. We have taken time to know what we want and how to go about it. We are now averaging 10 to 14 ambulatory surgeries a day, and I now feel we should be doing twice that. There are institutions that are doing more, although many of them are doing procedures that we as a Catholic hospital would not do. But we are fortunate to have an administration and a chief of surgery—Dr. O'Donovan and Dr. Carpenter—who believe in the value of this kind of service, believe in exploring all dimensions of the best way for us, and have cooperated completely as we have been feeling our way."

As Doctor Holt explained, initiating an Ambulatory Surgery program is not just as simple as deciding "we're going to have one. Let's get started." Many other factors are involved—changes in laboratory procedures, streamlining the Admitting process, educating the medical staff to the merits of the service, educating patients to the concept, learning to carefully identify the type of patient geared to this type of surgery.

A good Ambulatory Surgery Department must be carefully planned and efficiently structured to pull other effected departments into the total process of getting the patient in and out in one day, while rendering to that patient the same quality care he would have if he were admitted as an inpatient.

All hospitals—and certainly most patients—have a realistic view of the huge cost of health care these days. Newspaper articles, television commentators, magazines shout it. A comparison of costs of Ambulatory Surgery versus a two or three day hospital stay—a dollar and cent view—is one way to convey the benefits to all concerned of Mount Carmel's program.

George Chesbro, head of Accounting for the hospital, says that "hospital costs are 90 to 95 per cent of the total charges for a patient. If there are less hospital costs involved, the savings is to the patient, to the hospital, and to the insurance company. All in all it is a much more economic way to go."

The cost of a semi-private room at this hospital is now $97 dollars a day. That savings to the patient is immediate. There is also, says Mr. Chesbro, a different charge structure for Ambulatory Surgery patients, since many of the hospital's departments are not at all involved in his care—dietary, for example, and housekeeping and extended nursing care.

The charge for use of the operating room for the Ambulatory Surgery patient is $95 dollars for the first half hour and $25 dollars for each additional half hour. The average cost to the patient here is running about $120 dollars. For inpatient surgery the charge for the operating suite is $200 for the first hour, and $50 for every extra half hour. Higher inpatient costs come from a variety of reasons—more supplies used in the surgery process, lengthier use of the O.R., more back-up support, more sterilizing procedures.

For the short-stay surgical patient, again according to Mr. Chesbro, that $95 dollar fee also covers all pre-op and recovery room charges. For inpatient surgery these is a post-anesthesia recovery charge of $25 for the first half hour and $10 for each additional half hour. More intensified care is obviously needed with more complex surgery.

If the short-stay patient has a nurse-anesthetist, the charge is a flat fee of $40 for a general anesthetic, and $20 for a local anesthetic. The inpatient here is paying $60 for the first hour and $12 for each additional half hour.

But in addition to the saving in time and money, other advantages can be quickly identified, says Dr. Holt.

"A housewife with a family, for instance, can be back home in the same afternoon after a procedure such as a breast biopsy. She doesn't have to find a baby sitter to care for the children, at least not for more than a few hours. Nor does her husband have to take more than a day off from work—and not even that if she is accompanied to the hospital by another family member. She's back in her own home, in her own bed, and the psychological boon to quick recovery is much greater than if she were separated from them and worrying about them.

"At the hospital a bed is reserved and available for a more acutely ill patient, one who might be on our medically urgent admitting list who is waiting for that bed.

"And it has one third very important advantage. Ambulatory Surgery certainly cuts down apprehension for the patient. They don't have time to be too afraid. The very fact that they come and go in a day is a tension-reliever. It is unfortunate, but, so many patients get so much bad information about surgery. A short stay minimizes fear. ·

"As an added benefit, we hope this type of program will bring down insurance premiums, for the patient and for the hospital."

The decision to bring a patient in for Ambulatory Surgery is made by his own doctor. Good judgment is of primary importance here, Dr. Holt stresses. A doctor may have a patient who could reasonably have this type of procedure. But if that patient is emotionally overcharged, highly nervous, whose response cannot be reliably predicted, or who may not follow doctor's orders about refraining from food and drink, it is probably better to bring this kind of patient into the house.

If the doctor decides his patient is stable and can accept this kind of program as an advantage to be taken, he then calls the Admitting desk and also the surgical desk and asks to be scheduled. Forms are sent out to the patient to be filled in at home, and an admitting time set.

"We like more notice obviously," says Dr. Holt, "but we can arrange all this even two days ahead of the needed surgery."

Also the patient's physician can process the lab work through his office— blood-work for all patients, plus urinalysis for those getting a general anesthetic—but it is preferred that that be done in the hospital. The patient is asked to report a couple of hours before scheduled surgery to allow time for lab work. The surgeon and the anesthesiologist have decided in advance the type of anesthetic, and if pre-op medication is to be given. If the patient is relaxed, a pre-op medication will not be given at all.

"Patients," relates Dr. Holt, "may get a local, a general or some type of IV anesthetic. If we give a general anesthetic, we will certainly also start an IV.

"We should emphasize that every single precaution that is taken for the in-house surgical patient is taken for the ambulatory patient. We monitor them all during the surgery. We do the same surgical set-ups, use all the same staff. We absolutely take no short-cuts. In fact, if it is possible, we are even more careful, since not as much is known about that particular patient as it might be about an in-house patient."

After the surgical procedure, the patient is taken to a Recovery Room where he is closely watched. Patients who have taken a local anesthetic are ready to leave the hospital relatively quickly. Patients who have been given a general anesthetic stay longer and are closely watched. They do not leave the hospital until they are fully alert, all vital signs are stable, they are experiencing no dizzyness.

As an added precaution, no ambulatory patient can leave the hospital alone. They must be accompanied and driven home. When they leave, they are discharged both by their own physician and by the anesthesiologist. And they leave with precise information on recuperative care.

"We require that the patient be accompanied," explains Dr. Holt, "because some patients may have a little hangover effect from the anesthetic, and this is true of IV medications as well as a general anesthetic. Regardless of what they think about how well in control they are, we know they may not be as sharp as they normally would be. We definitely don't want them driving."

"Also as a service to patients, we try to define for them the length of the procedure they will be undergoing. There are variables, but we try to give them as close to the average as possible. And we try not to make them wait. The surgery schedule will vacillate a little, but Irene Ignaczak, who does the scheduling, keeps things moving along right on time. This also helps the patient to minimize apprehension."

Hospitals all over the country are going into the field of Ambulatory Surgery very rapidly, Dr. Holt says, most either having a department or planning one to initiate one.

"This hospital is here to serve the community. This is another important approach to saving time and money for families, and is also an efficient use of an existing facility in the hospital."

Mount Carmel's Ambulatory Surgery Committee consists of: Dr. Willard S. Holt, chairman, Dr. A. Alexander, Dr. L.B. Gariepy, Dr. D. Olson, Dr. A. Stefani, Dr. J. Wade, Patrick Bridenstine, administrative assistant, and Miss Irene Ignaczak, R.N.

In an article prepared for a professional journal on Ambulatory Surgery,

Thomas R. O'Donovan, Administrator of Mount Carmel stated that, according to current estimates, "one-third of all hospital operations could be performed on a same-day basis, saving our nation's health care delivery system several billion dollars a year."

Dr. O'Donovan went on to say, "As we approach the 1980's over one-half of our nation's hospitals have no program of ambulatory surgery.

"According to the American Hospital Association, 'many types of minor surgery do not require overnight hospitalization. Therefore, hospitals must plan and provide ambulatory surgical facilities so that, whenever appropriate, surgery can be performed on an outpatient basis, thereby reducing cost to the patient, the hospital, and the community, and assuring optimum use of inpatient beds.'

"There is no question of the importance of ambulatory surgery in medical care in modern day America."

Appendix I

Selected Bibliography

Ahlgren, E. W. "Pediatric Outpatient Anesthesia: A Four-Year Review." *Am J Dis Child* 126:36-40, Jul 1973.

Aimakhu, V. E. "Out-Patient or Hospital Day-Care for Minor Gynaecological Procedures." *Niger Med J* 3:37-9, Jan 1973.

"An Answer to the Surgical Waiting List?" *Lancet* 2:23-4, Jul 1, 1972.

Armitage, E. N.; Howat, J. M.; and Long, F. W. "Day-Surgery Programme for Children Incorporating Anaesthetic Outpatient Clinic." *Lancet* 2:21-3, Jul 5, 1975.

Atwell, J. D. "Paediatric Day-case Surgery in Southampton." *Nurs Times* 71:841-3, May 29, 1975.

Atwell, J. D.; Burn, J. M.; Dewar, A. K.; and Freeman, N. V. "Paediatric Day-Case Surgery." *Lancet* 2:895-7, Oct 20, 1973.

Baumgart, A. J., and Smith, E. M. "Day Care for Young Children Undergoing Surgery." *Nurs Clin North Am* 6:531-5, Sep 1971.

Beaton-Mamak, M. "All in a Day's Work: The Case for Ambulatory Surgery." *Dimens Health Serv* 51:42-4, Aug 1974.

Bell, A. "Day Surgery: A Concept of Care for the Pediatric Patient." *AORN J* 19:623-31, Mar 1974.

Bellinger, J. "Fiscal Effects of an Outpatient Surgery Program." Thesis, Duke University, Durham, North Carolina, 1972.

Berrill, T. H. "A Year in the Life of a Surgical Day Unit." *Br Med J* 4:348-9, Nov 11, 1972.

Blanken, G. E. "Surgical Operations in Short-Stay Hospitals." *Vital Health Stat Series* 13(18):1-46, Nov 1974.

Bloomfield, E. "Surgical Procedures in a Health Centre." *Nurs Times* 69:299-301, Mar 8, 1973.

"Blue Cross Policy on Free Standing Ambulatory Surgical Facilities." *Ill Med J* 143:1-2 (suppl) Jun 1973.

Bregande, B. J. "Modular Units Offer Design Flexibility." *Hospitals* 49:66-9, Oct 1, 1975.

Brophy, T. "Day Patient Care—Philosophy and Practicality." *Nat Hosp* (Australia) 18:22, Sep 1974.

California Hospital Association: *Outpatient Surgery In Hospitals.* Sacramento, California, California Hospital Association, 1974.

Calnan, J., and Martin, P. "Development and Practice of an Autonomous Minor Surgery Unit in a General Hospital." *Br Med J* 4:92-6, Oct 9, 1971.

Calwell, H. C. "Outpatient Surgery in Children." *Br Med J* 4:551, Dec 2, 1972.

"Can Outpatient Surgicenter Beat Blue Cross Veto?" *Hosp Pract* 6:150, 154-5, 157-8, Feb 1971.

Carroll, J. "JCAH Sets Standards for Surgery in a Non-Hospital Setting." *AORN J* 19:649-51, Mar 1974.

Clayton, S. G. and others: "Shortstay Gynaecology Ward." *The Lancet:* 1197-98, Nov 27, 1971.

Cloud, D. T.; Reed, W. A.; Ford, J. L.; Linkner, L. M.; Trump, D. S.; and Dorman, G. W. "The Surgicenter: A Fresh Concept in Outpatient Pediatric Surgery." *J Pediatr Surg* 7:206-12, Apr 1972.

Coakley, C. S., and Levy, M. L. "Anesthesia for Ambulatory Surgery." *J Arkansas Med Soc* 68:101-4, Aug 1971.

Cohen, D. D., and Dillon, J. B. "Anesthesia for Outpatient Surgery." *JAMA* 196:1114-6, Jun 27, 1966.

"Come-and-Go Surgery Sparks Controversy." *Am Med News* 14:1, passim, Nov 29, 1971.

Comper, A. "Ambulatory (outpatient) Surgicare Centers." *Surg Bus* 37:28-33, Oct 1974.

Condon, S. R. "Day-Time Hospital for Children." *Am J Nurs* 72:1431-3, Aug 1972.

Cooper, R. "Day-Surgery Centers Snip Away Red Tape, Put Clamp on Costs." *Wall Street J* 1, 10, Jan 23, 1976.

Craig, G. A. "Use of Day Beds in Gynaecology." *Br Med J* 4:348-9, Jun 27, 1970.

Crosby, D. L.; Griffith, G. H.; Jenkins, J. R.; Real, R.; Roberts, B. C.; and Forrest, A. P. M. "General Surgical Pre-Admission Clinic." *Br Med J* 3:157-9, July 15, 1972.

Crosby, R. W. "Faster Hospital Service: In and Out." *Med Econ* 44:65-71, Aug 7, 1967.

Crouch, B. L.; Ford, J. L.; and Reed, W. A. "The Surgical Center: Concept, Care, Cost in a Freestanding Facility." *Hosp Top* 49:69-72, 81, Dec 1971.

Davenport, H. T.; Shah, C. P.; and Robinson, G. C. "Day Surgery for Children." *Can Med Assoc J* 105:498-501, Sep 4, 1971.

Davis, J. "Ambulatory Surgical Care: Basic Concept and Review of 1,000 Patients." *Surgery* 73:483-5, Apr 1973.

Davis, J. E. "Ambulatory Surgery Saves Time, Money." *Hosp World* 1:18, Apr 1972.

Davis, J. E. "Day Surgery: A Viable Alternative." *AORN J* 19:641-7, Mar 1974.

Davis, J.E. "Inpatient Surgery on an Ambulatory Basis." *NC Med J* 34:356-9, May 1973.

Davis, J.E. "One Day Surgery." *Hosp Top* 52(42), April 1974.

Davis, J. E., and Detmer, D. E. "The Ambulatory Surgical Unit." *Ann Surg* 175:856-62, June 1972.

Dawe, C.L. "Outpatient Surger." *Australian Nurs J* J3(2): 26-28, Aug 1973.

Delany, H. M. "A Surgeon's View of a Community Health Center." *Surgery* 73:486-9, Apr 1973.

Diggory, P. "Outpatient Abortion." *Lancet* 2:767-8, Oct 2, 1971.

Doenicke, A.; Kugler, J.; and Laub, M. "Evaluation of Recovery and 'Street-fitness' by EEG and Psychodiagnostic Tests After Anesthesia." *Canadian Anaesth Soc J* 14: 567, 1967.

Doran, F. S.; White, M.; and Drury, M. "The Scope and Safety of Short-Stay Surgery in the Treatment of Groin Herniae and Varicose Veins. A report on 705 cases." *Br J Surg* 59:333-9, May 1972.

Downey, G. W. "Outpatient Surgery: If You Can't Beat It, Join It." *Mod Hosp* 120:88-9, June 1973.

Drury, M.; Doran, F. S.; and White, M. "Short-Stay Surgery and General Practice." *J R Coll Gen Pract* 23:55-8, Jan 1973.

Edelson, E. "New 'Come-and-Go Surgery.' " *Fam Health* 5:41-4, Sep 1973.

Editorial. "Tottering Home: The Matter of Outpatient Surgery." *Lancet* 1:1366-7, June 21, 1975.

Egdahl, R. H. "Ambulatory Health-Care Delivery and the Surgeon." *Surgery* 73:637-8, Apr 1973.

Epstein, B. S.; Coakley, C. S.; and Levy, M. L. "Outpatient Surgery." *Hospitals* 47:80-4, Sep 1, 1973.

Eyring, E. J. "Letter: Outpatient Orthopedic Procedures." *New Engl J Med* 290:633-4, Mar 14, 1974.

Fahy, A., and Marshall, M. "Postanaesthetic Morbidity in Out-Patients." *Br J Anaesth* 41:433-8, May 1969.

Feins, N. R. "Pediatric Surgery; Current Concepts." *Pediatr Clin North Am* 21:361-8, May 1974.

Ferguson, L. K. *Ferguson's Surgery of the Ambulatory Patient.* Edited by M. W. Wolcott. 5th ed. Philadelphia, J. B. Lippincott Company, 1974.

Floerchinger, J. "A Fight for the Right to Compete." *Private Pract* 5:46-54, Aug 1973.

Fogel, L. N. "Outpatient Presurgical Care Conserves Inpatient Days." *Hospitals* 43:51-4, Jan 1, 1969.

Ford, J. L., and Reed, W. A. "The Surgicenters. An Innovation in the Delivery of Medical Care." *Ariz Med* 26:801-4, Oct 1969.

Forsyth, G., and Logan, R. F. *Gateway or Dividing Line? A Study of Hospital Outpatients in the 1960's.* London, Oxford University Press, 1968.

"Free-Standing Surgical Center: A First for Texas." *Tex Med* 70:106-8, Mar 1974.

Funderburk, W. W. " 'In-and-out' Surgery Using General Anesthesia. A Personal Experience." *J Natl Med Assoc* 66:416-9, Sep 1974.

Gallese, L. R. "When Some People Tell About Operation, The Story is Short." *Wall Street J* 1, 15, Jan 4, 1974.

Gien, I. "Outpatient Surgery in Day Clinics." *S Afr Med J* 45:1395-7, Dec 18, 1971.

Goldberg, M. H., and Mark, H. I. "Anesthesia for the Dental and Surgical Out-Patient." *J Am Dent Assoc* 75:1376-8, Dec 1967.

Golditch, I. M., and Huston, J. E. "Therapeutic Abortion Without Inpatient Hospitalization." *Calif Med* 116:1-3, Mar 1972.

Green, M. "Innovative Methods of Expanding Ambulatory Services." *Adv Pediatr* 20:15-38, 1973

Haig, J. D., and Lambley, D. K. "A Work Study on a Surgical Out-Patient Clinic." *Hospital* (London) 61:522-4, Oct 1965.

Haley, T. M., and Keenan, W. L. "Surgery by Day, Home by Night, Savings All the Time." *Mod Hosp* 111:113, Sep 1968.

Hannon, F. "The Ambulatory Surgery Unit: Its Cost Feasibility, with Specific Reference to Rex Hospital, Raleigh, North Carolina." Unpublished Thesis. Duke University, Durham, North Carolina, 1973

Harmon, C. "Optimum Staffing Levels for the Watts Hospital Special Surgical Unit (SSU)." Unpublished Thesis. Duke University, Durham, North Carolina, 1973.

Hart, P. F. "Separate Service for Surgery Can Cut Hospital Admissions." *Hosp Admin Can* 9:90-1, Sep 1967.

Hart, P. F. "Surgical Day Care." *Hosp Admin Can* 13:68, 70, May 1971.

Hauff, W. R. "Case Study: Renovation and Expansion of Health Facilities: Centralized Outpatient Care." *Hospitals* 48:87-90, Feb 1, 1974.

Hawthorne, D. "Economy of Health Care Through the Effective Utilization of Day Surgery. Unpublished Thesis. Trinity University, San Antonio, Texas, 1972.

Hawthorne, D. "Hospital-Based Unit Improves Utilization." *Hospitals* 49:62-5, Oct 1, 1975.

Hendren, W. H. "Pediatric Surgery. 1." *N Engl J Med* 289:456-62, Aug 30, 1973.

Herzfeld, G. "Hernia in Infancy." *Amer J Surg* 39:422-29, 1938.

Hill, C. L. "Ambulatory Surgical Facility." *RI Med J* 58:313-4, Jul 1975.

Hill, C. L. "Ambulatory Surgical Facility—Concept is Consistent with Containment of Cost and Quality of Care." *RI Med J* 58(7):312-314, July 1975.

Hill, C. L. "Editorial: Medical Crises—The Elective Surgical Patient. *RI Med J* 52:429, 435, Aug 1969.

Hill, C. L. "Evolution of the Surgicenter." *RI Med J* 56:462-3, Nov 1973.

Hill, C. L. "Surgicenters." *RI Med J* 55:14-5, Jan 1972.

Hill, G. J. "Editorial: Outpatient Surgery—What are the Indications for It?" *Surgery* 77:333-5, Mar 1975.

Hill, G. J., (Ed.). *Outpatient Surgery.* Philadelphia, W. B. Saunders Company, 1973.

Hokr, W. K. "Anesthesia and the Mini-Surgicenter for Ambulatory Surgical Gynecology." *Clin Obstet Gynecol* 17(3):249-54, Sep 1974.

Holton, F. A. "Surgicenter: New Way to Cut Hospital Costs." *Physicians Manage* 11:23-9, Dec 1971.

Holton, F. A. "What Future Now for Surgical Centers?" *Prism* (Chicago) 3:46-8, 50-2, Mar 1975.

Horoshak, I. "Outpatient Surgery: R.N. Role Grows with the Field." *RN* 38:47, 50, 52-6, Jul 1975.

"Hospitals Should Meet Need for Outpatient Surgery." (News) *Mod Hosp* 121:33, Jul 1973.

"In and Out Surgery." *Perspective* 9:1-14, Third Quarter, 1974.

Irwin, T. "We Need More Same Day Surgical Centers." *Today's Health:* 10, Jan 1976.

Janis, K. M. "Hospital-Based Outpatient Anesthesia Service: Organization and Management." *Hosp Med Staff* 2:12-16, Feb 1973.

Jones, C. W. "Anesthesia for Outpatient Surgery." *J Natl Med Assoc* 66:411-5, Sep 1974.

Kernaghan, S. G. "Peripheral Issues Cloud Basic Questions in Day Surgery." *Hospitals* 49:58-61, Oct 1, 1975.

Kirkland, M. L. "Surgery Economics." *Amer Assoc Nurs Anesth* 43:48-53, Feb 1975.

Knapp, M. R.; Owen, P. A.; Owen, L. W.; Wallace, R.; and Clark, C. "Minor Surgery Center: An Answer to Escalating Costs." *J Kans Med Soc* 74:446-9, Dec 1973.

Kohlman, H. A. "Hospital is Proper Focal Point for Short-Stay Surgery." *Hosp Financ Manage* 28:22-4, Jun 1974.

Lahti, P. T. "Early Post-Operative Discharge." *Mich Med* 755-60, Sep 1970.

Lahti, P. T. "Early Post-Operative Discharge of Patients from the Hospital." *Surgery* 63:410-15, Mar 1968.

Lee, R. M. "Day Surgery has Added Benefits for Children." *AORN J* 19:632-5, Mar 1974.

Lee, R. M. "Standards Vital to Day Surgery Patient Care." *AORN J* 19:589-90, Mar 1974.

Leithauser, D. J., and Bergo, H. L. "Early Rising and Ambulatory Activity After Operation; Means of Preventing Complications." *Arch Surg* 42:1086-93, Jun 1941.

Levinson, J. M. "Outpatient Gynecological Surgery." *Del Med J* 42:258-60, passim, Oct 1970.

Levy, M. L., and Coakley, C. S. "Survey of In and Out Surgery—First Year." *South Med J* 61:995-8, Sep 1968.

Lewis, A. A. "Outpatient Surgery in a Developing Country." *Lancet* 1:910-2, Apr 19, 1975.

Lieb, L. "Health Care Challenges Demand New Solutions in the USA." *Surg Bus* 37:29-32, Jul 1974.

Lieberman, S. L.; Giacoia, E. B.; and Fedak, M. "Hospital-Based Outpatient Surgery. Anesthesia Experiences." *NY State J Med* 75:437-41, Feb 1975.

Lord, P. "Early Discharge from Hospital—The Consultant Surgeon's Point of View." *R Soc Health J* 92:297-9, Dec 1972.

Lynch, D. "Surgicenter Approach to Medicine." *Am Fam Physician* 3:141-4, Jun 1971.

McEwin, R. "Pre-Admission Clinics for Elective Surgery." *Hosp Health Admin* (Australia) 1:14-5, Nov-Dec 1971.

McIlroy, W. *A Day Surgery Program for Methodist Hospital, Dallas, Texas.* Unpublished Thesis. Baylor University, Waco, Texas, 1973.

McNerney, W. J. "How to Improve Medical Care: Interview with the Head of the Blue Cross Association. *US News World Rep* 66:42-6, Mar 24, 1969.

Maisel, A. Q. "How to Hold Down Rising Hospital Costs." *Readers Digest* 105:147-50, Nov 1974.

Markle, G. B., 4th "The Case for Doing More Office Surgery." *Med Econ* 51:75-9, Jan 7, 1974.

Markle, G. B., 4th "Letter: Ambulatory Surgical Unit." *Arch Surg* 109:124, Jul 1974.

Martin, P. L. "Ambulatory Surgical Gynecology: An Overview." *Clin Obstet Gynecol* 17(3):199-204, Sep 1974.

Martin, P. L., and Rust, J. A. "Surgical Gynecology for the Ambulatory Patient." *Clin Obstet Gynecol* 17(3):205-15, Sep 1974.

Morgan, D. "Humanization with Surgical Day Care." *Dimens Health Serv* 52:11-2, Jul 1972.

Morse, T. S. "Pediatric Outpatient Surgery." *J Pediatr Surg* 7:283-6, Jun-Jul 1972.

Nabatoff, R. A., and Stark, P. C. "Letter: Major Outpatient Surgery." *Lancet* 1:565-6, Mar 30, 1974.

Nagel, E. L.; Forster, R. K.; Jones, D. B.; and MacMahon, S. "Outpatient Anesthesia for Pediatric Ophthalmology." *Anesth Analg* (Cleveland) 52:558-61, Jul-Aug 1973.

Nagel, W. "Pallister Suite: Calgary's Mini-Hospital is Attracting Nationwide Attention." *Can Med Assoc J* 107:83-4, Jul 8, 1972.

Nathanson, B. N. "Ambulatory Abortion: Experience with 26,000 Cases (July 1, 1970 to August 1, 1971). *N Engl J Med* 286:403-7, Feb 24, 1972.

"New Centers for One-Day Surgery: Ambulatory Facilities Boom Due to Low Cost of Care." *Med World News* 16:65-6, Jan 27, 1975.

O'Donnell, W. E. "Ambulatory Patients Don't Belong in Hospitals!" *Med Econ* 51:157-8, passim, Dec 9, 1974.

O'Donovan, T. R. "Case for Ambulatory Short Stay Surgery." *Mich Hosp* 11:10-11, 22, Feb 1975.

O'Donovan, T. R. "Dynamics of Ambulatory Surgery." *Hosp Admin* (Chicago) 20:27-39, Win 1975.

O'Donovan, T. R. "Evaluation of the Factors that Tend to Differentiate Ambulatory Hospital Surgery from Independently Operated Freestanding Short-Stay Surgical Facilities." *Mich Hosp* 9:23, Jun 1973.

O'Donovan, T. R. "Future Trends in Ambulatory Short-Stay Surgery." *Dimens Health Serv* 51:40-1, Aug 1974.

O'Donovan, T. R. "Some Major Conclusions in Regard to Ambulatory Surgery in the United States." *Sinai Hosp Bulletin* 23(4):205-08, Oct 1975.

O'Donovan, T. R. "Ambulatory Surgery." *R Soc Health J,* London, England, published June 1976.

"One-Day Surgery: An Answer to Soaring Hospital Costs?" *Bus Week* No. 2388:62-3, Jul 7, 1975.

"One-Day Surgery: Instant Rivalry?" *Med World News* 13:39, passim, Mar 17, 1972.

"One-Day Surgery Is Spreading Fast." *US News World Rep* 74:50-1, May 28, 1973.

Othersen, H. B., Jr., and Clatworthy, H. W., Jr. "Outpatient Herniorrhaphy for Infants." *Am J Dis Child* 116:78-80, Jul 1968.

"Outpatient Clinic for Surgery; Facility Cuts Costs to Patients and Insurers." *Med World News* 12:58-9, Oct 8, 1971.

"Outpatient Operations." *Time Magazine* 101:57, Apr 2, 1973.

"Outpatient Surgery." *Hosp Admin Curr* 16:1-4, Apr 1972.

"Outpatient Surgery Units Successful, Well Accepted, Surgeons Report: Symposium." *Hosp Top* 50:46-51, Jul 1972.

Pent, D., and Loffer, F. D. "Laparoscopy as an Ambulatory Procedure." *Clin Obstet Gynecol* 17 (3):231-47, Sep 1974.

"Perform Minor Operations Successfully Out-of-Hospital." *Health Insurance News* p.1, May 1971.

"Phoenix' Surgicenter Takes 1972 Lambert Award." *Am Surg Dealer* 59:27-8, Dec 1972.

Pipicelli, T. P. "Cost Analysis of the Day Surgery Program at Middlesex Memorial Hospital." (M.S. Essay.) Presented to the Faculty of the Department of Epidemiology and Public Health, Yale University, New Haven, Connecticut, 1974.

Prioleau, W. H. "Surgery at the General Infirmary at Leeds Under the British Health System." *J SC Med Assoc* 70:369-372, Nov 1974.

Reed, W. A.; Crouch, B. L.; and Ford, J. L. "Anesthesia and Operations on Outpatients." *Clin Anesth* 10(3):336-56, 1974.

Reed, W. A., and Ford, J. L. "The Surgicenter: An Ambulatory Surgical Facility." *Clin Obstet Gynecol* 17(3):217-30, Sep 1974.

Reichman, S. "Challenge to Hospitals: Improve Ambulatory Care." *Hosp Med Staff* 3:31-7, May 1974.

"Report on the Phoenix Surgicenter." *Contemporary OB/Gyn* 3:119-128, May 1974.

Reynolds. J. A. "Why is In-and-Out Surgery Gathering Dust? At Issue: Health Planning, Politics, and Profits." *Med Econ* 52:163-5, 69-70, 72-4, May 12, 1975.

Rhu, H. S., and Rust, J. A. "Economics of Ambulatory Surgical Gynecology." *Clin Obstet Gynecol* 17(3)291-4, Sep 1974.

Richards, M. T. "Uterine Curettage as an Office Procedure." *Can Med Assoc J* 107:133-4, Jul 22, 1972.

Robertson, J. R. "Ambulatory Gynecologic Urology." *Clin Obstet Gynecol* 17(3):255-76, Sep 1974.

Rockwell, S. M. "Surgicenter Staff? It's 100% R.N.s and Here's Why." *RN* 35:or/er 1-2, Mar 1972.

Rockwell, S. M. "Surgicenter: The One-Day Surgical Facility." *RN* 35:33-9, Mar 1972.

Rogatz, P. "Excessive Hospitalization can be Cut Back." *Hospitals* 48:51-6 120, Aug 1, 1974.

Rosenberg, C. L. "A Short-Stay Surgical Center for Your Patients?" *Med Econ* 48:114-5, passim, Nov 8, 1971.

Rosoff, C. B. "Editorial: Controlling the Cost of Hospital Care." *Arch Surg* 108:141, Feb 1974.

Ruckley, C. V.; Ludgate, C. M.; MacLean, M.; and Espley, A. J. "Major Outpatient Surgery." *Lancet* 2:1193-6, Nov 24, 1973.

Ruckley, C. V.; Smith, A. N.; MacLean, M.; and Small, W. P. "Team Approach to Early Discharge and Outpatient Surgery." *Lancet* 1:177-80, Jan 23, 1971.

Rupnik, E. J.; Williams, E. L.; and Johnson, W. C. "Breast Biopsy. An Outpatient Procedure Using Local Anesthesia." *Milit Med* 133:743-7, Sep 1968.

Ryan, G. B. "Can Freestanding Surgical Centers and Hospitals Coexist?" *Mod Med* 43:22-7, May 1, 1975.

Saltzstein, E. C., and Sullivan, C. B. "Outpatient Surgery." *Wis Med J* 74:S57-9, May 1975.

Saltzstein, E. C.; Sullivan, C. B.; Patterson, E. M.; and Hiller, J. A. "Ambulatory Surgical Unit: Alternative to Hospitalization." *Arch Surg* 108:143-6, Feb 1974.

Schimmel, E. M. "The Hazards of Hospitalization." *Ann Intern Med* 60:100-10, Jan 1964.

Schneider, R. J. "A Comprehensive Study of Free-Standing Outpatient Surgical Facilities." Unpublished Master's Thesis. St. Louis University, St. Louis, Missouri, 1973.

Shaw, A. "Outpatient Repair of Hernias in Infants and Children." *Va Med Mon* 102:214-9, Mar 1975.

"Short-Stay Surgical Centers: A Statement by the California Medical Association Commission on Health Facilities." *Calif Med* 119:87, Aug 1973.

"Short-Stay Surgical Facilities: Hospital-Based or Freestanding?" *Bull Am Coll Surg* 57:30-1, Apr 1972.

Somers, A. R. "Only the Hospital Can Do It All—Now." *Mod Hosp* 119:95-8, 100, Jul 1972.

"Statement on Ambulatory Surgical and Single Procedure Facilities: American Hospital Association." *Hospitals* 47:132-3, Aug 1, 1973.

Stehling, L. C., and Zauder, H. L. "Outpatient Surgery." *Tex Med* 70:61-4, Aug 1974.

Steward, D. J. "Outpatient Pediatric Anesthesia." *Anesthesiology* 43:268-76, Aug 1975.

"String of Walk-In-Clinics in Midwest; Projects of Mediclinic Corp., Des Plaines, Ill." *Amer Surg Dealer* 61:32, passim, Dec 1974.

The Surgical Suite: Functional Programming Worksheets. DHEW Publication No. (HSM) 73-4004, U.S. Government Printing Office, Washington, D.C., 1973.

"Surgicenters—New Idea for One Day Surgery." *Resident Staff Physician* 19:1s-6s, Apr 1973.

Taylor, D. H. "Medical-Surgical Day Care Unit." *Am J Nurs* 73:2109-10, Dec 1973.

Thompson, G. E.; Remington, M. J.; Millman, B. S.; and Bridenbaugh, L. D. "Experiences with Outpatient Anesthesia." *Anesth Analg* (Cleveland) 52:881-7, Nov-Dec 1973.

Tisdale, B. "Not for Admission." *Can Nurs* 68:35-9, Dec 1972.

Treloar, E. J. "An Out-Patient Anaesthetic Service: Standards and Organization." *Can Anaesth Soc J* 14:596-604, Nov 1967.

"Walk-in Surgery." *Newsweek* 83:56, Jan 21, 1974.

Wann, S.; Kangas, D.; and Udvare, D. "Operating Room Nursing in a Freestanding Center." *AORN J* 19:636-40, Mar 1974.

Warner, R. C. "An Investigation into the Regulatory Control of the Surgical Facility." Unpublished Thesis. Department of Industrial Engineering, Texas A & M University, College Station, Texas, 1970.

"We're Practicing In-and-Out Surgery. It's Great!" *Med Econ* 52:175, 177, 180, passim, May 12, 1975.

Wilk, H. G. "An Analysis of the Physician's Decision for Performing Minor Inpatient Surgical Procedures on an Ambulatory (Day Care) Basis." Unpublished Master's Thesis. School of Public Health, University of California, Berkeley, California, 1972.

Wilson, W. E. "Preoperative Anxiety and Anesthesia: Their Relation." *Anesth Analg* (Cleveland) 48:605-11, Jul-Aug 1969.

Young, P. E. "Abortion and Menstrual Extraction for the Ambulatory Patient." *Clin Obstet Gynecol* 17(3):277-90, Sep 1974.

Index

About the Editor

Dr. Thomas R. O'Donovan has been the Administrator of Mount Carmel Mercy Hospital in Detroit, Michigan, since 1971. He began working at the hospital twelve years ago as Associate Administrator. He is the author of three books and nearly sixty articles. For some of his articles, he has received major editorial awards. Over the past ten years, Dr. O'Donovan has presented more than ninety speeches and papers in the health care field. He has been the National Chairman of the Education Council, American Academy of Medical Administrators since 1971.

He is a Fellow, American College of Hospital Administrators, American Academy of Medical Administrators, and Royal Society of Health.

Dr. O'Donovan was included in the 1967 edition of *Outstanding Young Men of America* and was the recipient of the AAMA award as Medical Administrator of the Year in 1971.